OBSESSION

OBSESSION

A History / LENNARD J. DAVIS

THE UNIVERSITY OF CHICAGO PRESS

Chicago and London

LENNARD J. DAVIS is professor in the departments of English,
Disability and Human Development, and Medical Education
at the University of Illinois at Chicago.

The University of Chicago Press, Chicago 60637
The University of Chicago Press, Ltd., London
© 2008 by Lennard J. Davis
All rights reserved. Published 2008
Printed in the United States of America

17 16 15 14 13 12 11 10 09 08   1 2 3 4 5

ISBN-13: 978-0-226-13782-7 (cloth)
ISBN-10: 0-226-13782-1 (cloth)

A portion of chapter 5 previously appeared in "Never Done: Compulsive
Writing, Graphomania, Bibliomania," *Fictions* 4 (2005). Chapter 8 was
previously published as "Play It Again, Sam, and Again: Obsession and
Art," *journal of visual culture* 5:2 (2006), 242–66.

Library of Congress Cataloging-in-Publication Data

Davis, Lennard J., 1949–
Obsession : a history / Lennard J. Davis.
p. ; cm.
Includes bibliographical references and index.
ISBN-13: 978-0-226-13782-7 (cloth : alk. paper)
ISBN-10: 0-226-13782-1 (cloth : alk. paper)
1. Obsessive-compulsive disorder—History. 2. Compulsive behavior—History. I. Title.
[DNLM: 1. Obsessive Behavior—history. 2. Compulsive Behavior—history. 3. History,
Modern 1601–. 4. Obsessive-Compulsive Disorder—history.
WM 11.1 D2620 2008]
RC533.D38 2008
616.85'227009—dc22
2008014361

Contents

v

Obsession in Our Time

OBSESSIVE ME

When I was around six or seven, I began to have thoughts about death and dying that I couldn't push out of my mind. I realized that I was mortal and would die. I'd lie in bed and panic, sweat, and thrash around wrestling with the inevitability of my personal demise. To get those thoughts out of my mind, I developed certain rituals. I would try to envision in my mind's eye a black kitten that I had actually earlier brought home and was allowed to keep only until nightfall. That mental image comforted me, as did the vision of a white and cleanly wrapped loaf of Silvercup bread, whose advertising campaign had no doubt made me feel the comfort of food and the safety of home. But mostly, I would lie in bed at night and look out my window at the apartment building next to mine. I decided that I had to count every single window that was illuminated, and once the thought occurred to me, I began to do it compulsively. Since the building was substantial, the count took a fair amount of time. After I had arrived at a total number of illuminated windows, I would begin to doubt whether I had counted correctly. I would then recount. Then it would occur to me that someone might have turned their lights on or off. So another recount was necessary. I did this for hours until I was exhausted.

In the morning my mother worried about the dark circles under my eyes. I assured her everything was fine, since it would be pointless to explain what I had been doing and thinking. On the way to school, I might hit my shoe against a curb by mistake, so of course I had to scuff the other shoe to keep things symmetrical. When I arrived at the traffic light, I had a formula I had to say to myself—"I defy justice. Light change!"—over and over again until the light changed. I also had a compulsion to swallow coins, mostly pennies and dimes, but there were the nickels as well, which I did on a regular basis, with the subsequent visual delight of seeing these gleaming circles emerge from me shiny and cleaned by the acid of my digestive system. When I ate elbow macaroni, I would slide each elbow on the tine of a fork, so that the utensil contained four straightened tubes of pasta, and then I would swallow each one whole. Continuing on the culinary front, I divided my food into absolute and irrevocable sections that must never mix or touch one another. Also, in eating mashed potatoes or any moldable foods, I would create a circle, divide it into four quadrants, eat one quadrant, and then completely remake the food into a slightly smaller circle. And then I would repeat the whole process, as the circle got asymptotically smaller and smaller. In illustrating Zeno's paradox three dimensionally with my food, I was always satisfied, and endlessly caught in my web of complex rituals.

While I was doing that, my father and brother were compulsively washing their hands and surviving through their own developed rituals. Every night my father checked and rechecked the locks on the doors, the faucets, and gas jets while closing and rechecking all the kitchen cabinets, accompanied all the while by repetitive throat clearings and nasal sniffles. My brother lathered himself up so much that he eventually developed a skin rash. My mother was strangely untouched by all these machinations. In the 1950s and in an immigrant, working-class, and under-educated family, we didn't have a name for these kinds of activities. We didn't know we were engaged in obsessional and compulsive activities. We were just doing what came naturally to us in our time and place.

OBSESSIVE YOU

I am sure as I write these words that countless people all over the country are doing similar things. They are engaged in obsessive-compulsive activities like cleaning and checking, fighting off intrusive thoughts, addictively thinking about sex, food, alcohol, drugs as well as acting on these addictions. People are also working at their jobs addictively and obsessively and then playing hard in an extension of their workday. Many folks are addicted to their nightly television shows, to collecting things, or to obsessing about that someone who is unattainable or lost forever. And not only people, but also our pets are engaged in such activities, as a recent issue of *Cat Fancy* magazine suggests in its cover story "Is This Normal? Recognize Your Cat's Obsessive Behavior."

Indeed, we live in an age of obsession; or more to the point, an age that is obsessed with obsession. No hot romance movie is complete without the idea that the lovers are obsessed. No scientist or musician's reputation is safe without the word "obsessed" tacked to his or her occupation. A perfume seductively carries the name. Talk-show listeners describe themselves as addicted to twenty-four-hour news and discussion. A *New York Times Magazine* special supplement on people obsessed with home design began with a surprising confession from the editor—"You're probably not going to believe this, but I don't have an obsession. . . . I may not be obsessed, but I'm grateful for those who are."[1] As the editor pointed out, "Obsession is a commitment; you have to believe in it, because it soon takes you over." To be without an obsession is, according to this view, something extraordinary. The article focuses on "three of the obsessives who are featured in this issue. If the others are working on a smaller scale, no matter. Their passions are just as grand, and their stories just as compelling."

At the beginning of the twenty-first century, obsession is seen both as a dreaded disease and as a noble and necessary endeavor. And that is the point of this book. How can a disease also be, when you use a different lens, a cultural goal? Another way of asking this question is, can a disease have a biography? Can there be a genealogy of collective and personal behaviors? How did we get to the point where our diseases are our obsessions and our obsessions are our diseases?

THE DARK SIDE

Obsession can be a cultural trait devoutly to be wished, but it also has a darker side. When I mention obsession to most people, I get a nudge and a wink. They assume that I am really talking about the kinky world of the erotic. Indeed, obsession has a kind of poetic darkness written into its phonemes, and a quick tour of the library catalog will produce a welter of fiction with suggestive titles like *Dark Obsession, Murder and Obsession, Deadly Obsession, A Haunting Obsession, Secret Obsession, Passionate Obsession, Intimate Obsession,* and so on. In the world of the erotic, obsessions have their special place. Some might claim that love isn't love unless it is obsessive. One author of a book on the subject writes,

> I should make it clear that I am talking about one particular kind of love: romantic, obsessive love, the hot thing we fall into, the love we're all expected to experience and that we call true love. Think of novels like *Wuthering Heights* and *Dr. Zhivago,* or films like *Casablanca* and *The English Patient.* . . . What they have in common is this: two people obsessed with each other while all the ordinariness of life, its consolations and diversions, vanishes.[2]

An entire range of literature and film is devoted to the proposition that in the world of relationships no obsession should go untried. With handcuffs, leather, whips, hot wax, toys, oils, latex and leather jumpsuits, nudity, and blindfolds, sex—anal, oral, acrobatic, submerged, drugged, drunk, gay, multipartnered, dangerous, anonymous—seems to need obsessions. This true, hot love is contrasted with the domestic mundane love of ordinary people—sexual convolutions versus Mom and Pop missionary alignments. In order to have a Heathcliff and Cathy or a Humbert and Lolita, you need to have an Ozzie and Harriet or the Waltons providing a baseline of nonobsessive, companionate couplehood. And mere affection pales by comparison with stalking-induced rapture.

Obsessive love is dangerous, and in fiction often leads to murder and mayhem. Yet it provides a kind of fantasy standard that advertising and commercial interests need to promote. The idea behind the product so advertised is that it will provoke in others an obsessive desire for one's own too well known and unexceptional body. The aura of the obsessive hovers over one's ordinary flesh like a mirage of desire over a parched desert. A Gallup Poll analysis of the ad campaign for Calvin Klein's perfume Obsession turned up the reaction of one consumer who said, "Use Obsession for a great sex life? I used it and nothing happened. I'm not having a great sex life."[3] This reader needed obsession either in herself or those within sniffing distance of her. Products like these ask us whether we can bear to live lives of quiet respiration devoid of infatuated chaleur.

We live in a culture that wants its love affairs obsessive, its artists obsessed, its genius fixated, its music driven, its athletes devoted. We're told

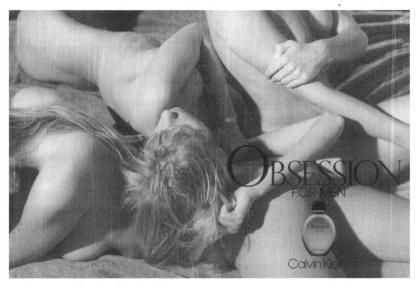

FIGURE 1. Calvin Klein Obsession ad.

that without the intensity provided by an obsession things are only done by halves. Our standards need to be extreme, our outcomes intense. Winners never quit and quitters never win. Emily Martin has recently shown how even corporations are trying to exploit the energy and focus of aberrant mental states, like obsession, for their own purposes.[4] Obsessives play obsessively on the streets, in the bars, and in the clubs, stay late in the offices, crank out the articles, novels, books, music, and films of our driven culture. To be obsessive is to be American, to be modern.

THINKING OBSESSION THROUGH

It is then perhaps coincident that obsessive-compulsive disorder rose to greater public attention in the 1990s, becoming one of the dominant forms of mental distress. A cavalcade of books on OCD have appeared in the past ten years, along with more books on antidepressants like Prozac and their use with OCD. More and more characters in television shows and film are people with OCD. In addition, anorexia, bulimia, and other obsessive and compulsive behaviors, like addiction, stalking, compulsive shopping, compulsive eating (or noneating) are plaguing and at the same time defining us. These are the other darker sides of obsession—the rooted-in-the-blood, bone, and mind forms of the fascination our culture has for the obsessive.

But was it always this way? The aim of this book is to show us how we got to this state of affairs—how it is that obsession now defines our culture. It is easy to say that people have always been obsessed or that the desire to find something and focus on it is a universal feature of human life. You couldn't build the pyramids or come up with *The Iliad* unless someone were obsessed enough to do so. True enough, but there is a moment in the Western world when obsession becomes itself something so problematic that people begin to write about it, study it, turn it into a medical problem, and then try to cure it. That defining moment, beginning in the middle of the eighteenth century in England and France, is worth looking at. Before that divide, some people were seen either as eccentrics, or in a more religious mode as "possessed." After that time, the age of obsession begins as a secular, medical phenomenon.

It may be objected that what I've just highlighted isn't obsession in a psychiatric sense, but more properly concerns an interest, a preoccupation, a fixation, or perhaps just a hobby. Indeed, in recent lectures I have given to psychotherapists, psychiatrists, and psychoanalysts, several objected that I was using the term "obsession" in a rather loose way. One insisted that the notion of an obsession, from a psychoanalytic perspective, was specifically about a recurring thought whose content had become disconnected from its original significance while the repetitive, recurring mental intrusion had come to predominate. Another found himself very irritated with me, saying that I was confusing a cultural activity with a brain-induced, life-and-death issue, and that he himself had a patient with OCD who might die within a few weeks. How could I equate a perfume with this kind of real suffering?

So I want to say now very clearly that I am not denying the existence of OCD as a disease. I follow the lead of the discussions of whether a disease is "real" or not from the work of Ian Hacking and Charles E. Rosenberg, among others.[5] Hacking recounts the many psychiatric disorders that come and go over time, and he says that the question of whether an illness is actually real doesn't fully do justice to the complexity of the situation. The assumption of the realness of a disease is taken out of any worldly or societal context. The assumption is that if a doctor and a patient elaborate a disease entity, then it isn't real. But scholars like Rosenberg emphasize that "a time- and place-specific repertoire of such agreed-upon disease categories has, in fact, always linked laypersons and medical practitioners and thus has served to legitimate and explain the physician's status and healing practice."[6] I have no doubt that OCD is real to people suffering from it and real to doctors trying to help those people. I also have no doubt that the search for a biological basis for OCD is a real search that aims to find specific brain functions, chemical interactions, and genetic locations that can help us understand how OCD manifests itself. But none of that prevents us from asking how certain behaviors came to be linked to a disease, how a society at large can influence which behaviors are seen as symptoms, and how researchers arrived at their own ways of organizing knowledge and developing protocols. Our problem comes when we try to deny that diagnosis is a complex process that aims to freeze in a moment the moving target of individual bodies and their processes interacting with psyches, environments, and social, institutional, and cultural milieus. In other words, OCD is real, and so are the circumstances that surround it and bring it into our clinical and social focus.

To make this point a little clearer, let's think about money. Money isn't a naturally occurring thing. It is a totally human-made invention, and yet it is real. Its rules are socially constructed, and its effects can be radical. People without money suffer in a real way. Economists can study how money circulates and gains or loses value. It is a genuine object of study, but it is completely socially constructed. It exists physically in the world, but it also has a symbolic existence. If you hold expired currency, it is still real, but it has lost its value by an abstract process. In asking whether money is real or not, we miss the point. Likewise disease. Disease exists to the extent that humans identify it and learn how it works. That learning can be of a medical kind, and that learning can extend to many other areas, from theoretical to common sense. I will talk more about how we come to know a disease, particularly a psychiatric disease, but I want to make clear at this point that the old saws of "nature or nurture" and "real or constructed" are not the ones I want to be hewing with right now.

CATEGORIZING OBSESSION

Psychiatrists take their definition of obsession from the *DSM-IV TR,* the diagnostic manual used by practitioners to define and categorize affective and cognitive conditions. obsessive-compulsive disorder is listed as one of several anxiety disorders. Its diagnostic number is 300.3, and it is described in this way:

> OCD is characterized by uncontrollable intrusive thoughts and action that can only be alleviated by patterns of rigid and ceremonial behavior. Symptoms frequently cause considerable distress and interference with daily social or work activities. There may be a major preoccupation with the smallest of details in daily life. Obsessive ideas frequently involve contamination, dirt, diseases, germs, real/imagined trauma, or some type of frightening/unpleasant theme. People recognize their obsessive ideas do not make sense but are unable to stop them. These obsessive thoughts frequently lead to compulsive behaviors as the person tries to prevent or change some dreaded event. They frequently repeat activities over and over again. (E.g., washing hands, cleaning things up, checking locks.)[7]

In making this type of definition, the common practice is to separate obsessions (thoughts) from compulsions (actions). To complicate the definition a bit further, there is also something called "obsessive-compulsive personality disorder," which is distinguished from the anxiety disorders. Its diagnostic number is 301.4, and it is described this way:

> Obsessive-Compulsive Personality Disorder is characterized by perfectionism and inflexibility. A person with an Obsessive-Compulsive Personality becomes preoccupied with uncontrollable patterns of thought and action. Symptoms may cause extreme distress and interfere with a person's occupational and social functioning.[8]

The former (OCD) is characterized by anxiety, while the latter is not a disorder but a personality type who may function quite well without anxiety or distress. If you have OCD, you do or think things you don't like doing, which makes you unhappy or distressed. If you have an obsessive-compulsive personality disorder, you may do the same things, but you may not mind. In fact, you may like doing or thinking such things.[9]

These are the types of categories concerning obsession that clinicians and practitioners use. Their definitions are useful to them as people whose job it is to diagnose and help cure people who present themselves as suffering from the obsessions and compulsions that are now called OCD. Indeed, one of the stated purposes of the *DSM* is to foster agreement among practitioners by providing common diagnostic categories. I don't wish to deny the utility of such descriptions or the benefits of the cures that have been developed. But I do wish to challenge what we might call the professional jurisdiction over the term "obsession." In some sense, the function of this book is to provide the broadest historical and cultural account of obsession to help explain how clinicians got to their profession-specific definition—how the split arose between the undesirable disease and the desirable cultural goal, between the formation of a pathological entity and the coming to be of a desired and necessary trait.

One could say more about obsessions as they are described clinically. There are obsessional thoughts, impulses, and images. Examples of obsessional thoughts are "Did I kill the old lady?" "Christ was a bastard." "Do I have cancer?" Obsessional impulses include: "I might expose my genitals in public." "I am about to shout obscenities in public." "I feel I might strangle a child." Unwanted obsessive images could include mutilated corpses, decomposing fetuses, a family member involved in a serious accident, unconventional sex with an unlikely person. One study ranked the content of obsessional material into five broad categories in order of frequency: dirt and contamination, aggression, orderliness of inanimate objects, sex, and religion.[10] Obsessive thoughts, according to one expert, fall into three main themes—aggressive, sexual, and blasphemous.[11] Another analysis lists "contamination, pathologic doubt, aggressive and sexual thoughts, somatic concerns, and the need for symmetry and precision."[12] Compulsions fall into three major categories—cleaning, checking, and counting.

OBSESSION AS CULTURE?

What I have just presented is the clinical definition of obsession, but it hardly accounts for what I hope to show is a continuing and serious cultural, historical, and social continuum. That is not to say that the clinical definition is not of interest to us all and does not provide us with a somewhat clear set of guidelines for choosing a particular kind of diagnosis and treatment. Indeed, some practitioners are willing to see connections between the clinical and the popular, as do Stanley Rachman and Ray Hodgson, who write that the popular usage of obsession "retains its utility."[13] What interests me in this project, therefore, moves beyond the desire to diagnose a patient and develop a set of treatments for that patient, which are necessary and valuable activities. Rather, I am more interested in how it came to be that someone on one side of the desk gets to perform a series of judgments and activities and the person on the other side of the desk gets to accede to those judgments and activities when both can be said to be obsessive. Or rather, how does the collaboration go on between the self-reporting patient and the category-giving doctor? In this particular case, one could argue that the physician who uses the *DSM-IV TR* is himself or herself using an obsessive text (obsessive in the sense of taxonomic and categorical—but more on that later)[14] to study with a single-minded fixation the patient who displays obsessive behavior.

As to the objection from clinicians that what I am talking about is not really OCD but more in the line of what one might call a focused activity, an idée fixe or simply a preoccupation, let me agree in the largest sense. But that distinction is also what I want to consider. I am interested in what makes a particular human activity worthy of study by other humans. I will argue, later in the work, that the kind of behavior that the eighteenth century regarded as eccentricity, curiosity, or fascination became, in a rather short period, something that split off into two parallel activities. One was the behavior, and the other was the study of the behavior. In other words, obsession became an illness, and the obsessive study of obsession became a profession. As this split happened, medicine—notably psychiatry and neurology—came into its own, and part of its professional agenda was the establishment of taxonomies and categories whose effect it was to separate out varieties of behavior into a signifying group of the pathological on the one hand and the heuristic on the other.

FINE DISTINCTIONS

It will be reasonable, at this point, to object to several things. Am I really saying that there is no difference between a man who cannot stop thinking about sheep and a man who intently studies the physiology of sheep? Is the man who must touch every lamppost really the same as the worker in an automobile assembly line who must paint every door that goes by him? Is a mother who worries obsessively about the safety of her child the same as a mother who just worries about her child? Surely there is a matter of degree, and in the case of the pathological, also a matter of logic. It makes sense to worry about your child, but it doesn't make sense to worry all the time about your child, especially when the child is asleep in the next room.

Of course it is foolish to think that all of these kinds of activities and thought patterns are the same. One wants to make distinctions, to separate the pathological from the normal. But if we simply accede to the reasonableness of the previous sentence, are we unthinkingly signing on to a kind of *doxa*? In my earlier book on the development of the concept of normality I raised questions about the obviousness of the normal.[15] Here, too, I want us to think about the way that human life gets sorted out into categories. Take, for example, the previously stated commonplace distinction between compulsions and obsessions. The *DSM-IV TR* makes a clear distinction. Obsessions are defined as "thoughts or impulses that are distressful, persistent and recurrent. These thoughts or impulses must not just be worries of real-life problems. The person must be aware that these thoughts or impulses are only a product of his/her own mind and they must be actively trying to suppress, ignore, or neutralize them with other actions." Compulsions "must show repetitive behavior, physical or mental, that cannot be controlled. (E.g., washing hands, checking locks, praying over and over again, counting or saying words repeatedly.) These actions must be aimed at trying to prevent or reduce some distressful situation."

The neat distinction between actions and thoughts are of course not as neat as they seem. Even the definition of compulsions includes the notion of "repetitive behavior, physical or mental." Mental behavior, in this case, includes praying, counting, or saying words mentally, that is, a kind of action within consciousness. But then, is thinking a nonmental activity? Is thinking a kind of mental doing? The fact that very few people have compulsions (only 9 percent in one study of obsessives) indicates that the neat line between obsession and compulsion has more to do with diagnostic categories than it might seem.[16] And obsessions can loop back into compulsions and vice versa, notably, for example, the obsession of doubting following the compulsive act of checking. I make this quibble because I want to highlight the fixation or infatuation behind the seemingly clear and neutral diagnostic criteria. But further, the demarcation between normal behavior and clinical categories is sometimes hard to determine. As Rachman and Hodgson note, "no one has offered a systematic statement of the necessary and sufficient conditions for deciding when and whether a reported experience is an obsession and when and whether a behavioral pattern should be described as compulsive."[17]

THE PROBLEM OF OBSESSION

This work has a complex and difficult set of aims. On a simple level, it is an attempt to describe the history of a disorder that was often considered a disease. But I think it is important to understand that no disease exists outside its cultural context. Even cholera, the gold standard for a "real" disease, means one thing in one culture and another in a different culture. Susan Sontag has shown us that disease is about metaphors.[18] So thinking of obsession as simply a disease is a mistake. Obsession is something that becomes a problem for Western culture at a certain moment in history—a problem because it is both the object of study and the way that we study that object. As with the problem of the mind—you can't study the mind with the mind—obsessive investigation of obsessive activity is bound to run into a problem. Our dilemma with obsession— our need for it and our fear of it—is a result of a series of unresolved issues that has haunted our culture since the middle of the eighteenth century.

The simple point of this work is that our obsession with obsession didn't just appear during our own time. This is a fascination and/or a disease that has a history. So this work fits into the larger project of the social history of medicine. But obsession isn't simply a medical category; it is a category of existence. There are obsessives, and there is obsession. Obsessives, if their obsessions are too obsessive, will be treated by medical doctors, particularly if they happen to be born after 1850; if not too obsessive, they will be humored or even admired. In saying that the problem isn't solely medical, I am saying that it is *biocultural.* That term, coined by David Morris, and expanded upon by others, including myself, is used to call into question the range of occurrences, experiments, statements, and discourses that have worked in the past by bracketing science on the one side and the humanities on the other. The goal of a biocultural project is to redeploy culture into the sciences and medicine so that a new synergy and wholeness can illuminate these complex projects.[19]

BIOCULTURAL VIEW OF OBSESSION

One must not take a phenomenon like OCD in isolation. The danger of a clinical perspective is that it tends to define the disease entity in universal terms, such that a patient with a particular disease will have these particular symptoms and outcomes in all situations at all times. But in the case of obsessive activity, one wants to begin to see how the activity fits into cultural paradigms and even into the same paradigms that the practitioner uses for observation, diagnosis, and treatment. To construct an artificial discontinuity between practitioner and patient is to fall into a kind of fallacy generated by the observational mechanism itself. Take for example the characteristics of a compulsive activity as described by Rachman and Hodgson: "precise . . . repetitive, unchanging, mechanical behavior."[20] The first question one might want to pose is, how much of such behavior is a result of a transformed culture?

One begins to see obsessional behavior as a cultural problematic that starts with modernity. This isn't to say that such behavior did not exist before, but it was not seen as problematic before except in the major area of religion. Religious scrupulosity and obsessive thoughts were more clearly problems for earlier times, although the medicalization of scrupulosity is of very recent occurrence.[21] Obsessive thoughts were more clearly tied to possession by the devil until the end of the seventeenth century when, at least in England, demonic possession was legally banned, since it was seen as tied up with Catholicism and popery. So, by the time the eighteenth-century man of letters Samuel Johnson walked down the street touching every light post, his peers noted the behavior and thought it was eccentric but without further consequence. No one called an exorcist. Yet almost a hundred years later when Macaulay noted Johnson's behavior, he saw it as part of a pattern of insanity. And now in the twenty-first century, when clinicians talk about Dr. Johnson, they retrospectively diagnose him as having Tourette syndrome. Each of these eras, including our own, felt they had the explanation down pat.

When an industrial culture evolves to emphasize and rely on a greater sense of precision, repetition, standardization, and mechanization, that same culture will perhaps regard those attributes differently, and members of that society will mime, imitate, embody, internalize, and exaggerate those qualities. Likewise, those members who called themselves scientists might well engage in those behaviors and focus their gaze on what they perceive as aberrations of such behavior. Take for example the following description of attempts to classify obsessional behavior:

> Kringlen . . . reported that over 50 per cent of the 91 obsessional patients included in his series complained of phobic symptoms. Kringlen subdi-

vided the obsessional patients into four categories and concluded that one-third of the group had a mixture of obsessional thoughts, acts, and phobias while 19 per cent had "predominantly or solely phobias." The stability of the phobic symptoms is attested to by the fact that when the follow-up investigation was carried out, an average of 16 years after admission to the hospital, no less than 69 per cent of the remaining 84 patients complained of phobic symptoms.[22]

Of course this is the quantified language of science and research, but one notes what we might call the obsessive use of numbers in repetition, which provide a patina of incontrovertibility and learning to a discourse that is characterized by its single-minded focus on a specific group of people—obsessives.[23]

OBSESSION AS MODERN CONSCIOUSNESS

Rachman and Hodgson note that the criteria for thinking of behavior as compulsive is "an experienced sense of pressure" and an accompanying sense of "unwillingness to comply," since without the latter, the person would not have a sense that he or she indeed had a problem. For an idea, impulse, or image there is needed intrusiveness, internal attribution, unwantedness, and difficulty of control.[24] This would mean that the person could not keep the idea out of his or her consciousness, realized that the idea was coming from his or her own mind, didn't want the idea to keep arising, yet could not control the idea.

One thing that is striking about this set of conditions is how closely it compares with Michel Foucault's notion of societal control of individuals. Foucault elaborates on a transition in the eighteenth century from a society that controls externally through the use of direct force to one that controls by internalized self-regulation. Could we perhaps see obsession as the visible end of a regulatory mechanism gone wrong? Indeed, the internalization of societal rules, especially when it had been accompanied by the decline of a religious structure that might include mechanisms, like confession or expiation, could indeed cause a kind of massive, cultural building up of a collective superego, as it were. Rachman notes that what makes thoughts, often occurring to most people, obsessive comes with the labeling of those thoughts as repugnant and unacceptable:

Patients afflicted by recurrent obsessions commonly attach exaggerated significance to these thoughts and regard them as horrific, repugnant, threatening, dangerous. . . . Various patients have described their obsessional
thoughts, impulses, or images as: immoral, sinful disgusting, revealing, dangerous, threatening, alarming, predictive, insane, bewildering, and criminal. At a higher level, they interpreted these thoughts, impulses, or images
as revealing important but usually hidden elements in their character, such
as: these obsessions mean that deep down I am an evil person; I am dangerous; I am unreliable; I may become totally uncontrollable . . . ; I am weird,
I am going insane (and will lose control?); I am a sinful person; I am fundamentally immoral.[25]

While it is possible to describe this list in various ways, it is perhaps tempt-
ing to think of it as a taxonomy of modern consciousness. People in the past
may well have had these feelings and sensations, but there does seem to
be something uniquely contemporary about the litany of self-accusations.
Although Foucault never discussed the internal psychological mechanism
by which the process of self-regulation occurred, it is possible for us to
raise the point that the mechanism might look a lot like the obsessive-
compulsive motor we have been describing. We might think of the nineteenth century in Europe as rapidly reformulating its rules for behavior
and thought. Science and medicine provided a venue for this reformulation, and theories of eugenics, degeneration, evolution, and so on created
new and hierarchical categories of the human based on biometrics and
psychometrics. Racialized, nationalized, eugenicized, and gendered theories singled out the "good" and the "bad" in human behavior and mental-
ity. As the bar was raised on what the self was and how it should behave,
as the scientific gaze framed and measured the desired norms, deviation,
whether physical or mental, took on the guilty pallor of transgression.
Given this raising of the bar, we can speculate that a culture of obsession
began to develop, perhaps as a secular concept of "unwanted" or "repugnant" thoughts and feelings were inscribed into the societal narrative.
Nineteenth-century literature, art, and culture were filled with accounts
of obsessive behavior— seen as both unacceptable and yet typical of the
human condition. Raskolnikov, Bartleby, Kurtz, Dupin, Sherlock Holmes,
and Ahab, to name only a few, became cultural icons of the dangers and
attractions of obsessive acts and ways of being. Freud, then, could be seen

as simply someone who laid bare the problem that was more or less obvious to everyone—the reality that obsessive behavior was the underlying substrate of neurosis. Freud simply obsessed about obsessives, as we will later see.

DIRT, SEX, BLASPHEMY, VIOLENCE

When we consider the content of obsessions and compulsive activities we have some more clues to the societal element in the constellation.[26] Obsessional thoughts are, according to one study, primarily focused on dirt and contamination (59 percent of cases in one study), followed by aggressive thoughts around homicide or suicide (25 percent), impersonal/orderliness (23 percent), religion (9 percent). Sexuality, which one would assume was a big issue for obsessive activity, was rated as uncommon in one study and at 9 percent in another.[27] A more recent study indicates that one fourth of people with OCD had sexual obsessions within their lifetime, but in any current moment 13.3 percent had such obsessions.[28] Another study sees contamination in the obsessions of 45 percent of patients, repetitive doubts in 42 percent, somatic obsessions in 36 percent, need for symmetry in 31 percent, aggressive impulses in 28 percent, and repeated sexual imagery in 26 percent.[29] For compulsive activities, the most common are activities related to cleaning and checking. Contrary to the psychoanalytic perspective, which sees the particular obsession as a distraction from the central psychodynamic conflict, we might hope to glean some reasons why these particular activities are so common. Is there a reason why cleaning is the most frequent activity?

Cleaning is very often related to fears of contamination—whether through spreading germs or making contact with chemicals. Checking is by and large an act of securing oneself or family members against some danger. Cleanliness and security then are the aims of the majority of compulsive activities. One could argue that it is only with the development of the germ theory and an awareness of toxic chemicals in the environment that one could have developed the kind of contagious fear that motivates a compulsive cleaner. Likewise, only with some idea of domestic security, the creation of a special firewall between inside and outside, and with the advent of modern conveniences and dangers (like gas, electricity, pollutants, chemicals, computers, identity theft, and so on) could checking become a useful and then irrational activity. In other words, a certain set of societal and cultural preconditions are necessary, and an accompanying sense of protecting oneself or family, in order for those activities to be highlighted and themselves worried about. In fact, as I will mention later, worrying itself, as indicated by the use of the word "worry" in the modern sense, came into the English language during the nineteenth century.

Another area of note in obsessive behavior is what is called "primary slowness." This type of behavior is one in which a person will take an enormously long time to perform an activity like dressing, performing a household chore, or getting ready to go out. Of course, such slowness must be placed in comparison with other kinds of cultural activities. In a culture defined by speed, efficiency, and multitasking, primary slowness is in fact contrary to the very pulse and tone of modernity. When George Beard invented the concept of neurasthenia in the nineteenth century, he saw it as a disease in which weakness and enervation resulted from the fast-paced existence of modern life—the new sense of speed created by the railway, the telegraph, industrialization, and urban life. The aim of people like Frederick Taylor, who applied time and motion studies to the factory floor, was to speed up the lapidary and casual slowness of traditional workers, bringing them up to the rapid pace of the machine age. Primary slowness incorporates an awareness of this uptick in pacing, acting as a shocking counterpoint to the speed of modern life. However, in its deliberateness and aim at perfection, an aim also incorporated into the compulsive activity of cleaning and checking which seeks to eliminate any doubt or anomaly in the environment, primary slowness also serves the notion of perfectibility in modernity. If you get it slowed down enough, you can finally get it right. Indeed, nineteenth-century ideas of progress, eugenics, and civilization are unimaginable without an ethos of perfectibility.

NORMALITY AND OBSESSION

The line between normality and obsession is one of the most interesting aspects of this study. In a way, the diagnostician must create a firewall between normality and pathology in order to develop a set of tools and treatments. Where this firewall shows up is in the *DSM-IV TR* distinction between OCD and obsessive personality disorder. In the former, a set of behaviors interferes with the quality of a life. In the latter, people have an obsessive personality with rigid components, but they are generally happy with themselves and their lives. The difference between these two diagnoses disappears in the area of insight and compliance. The rigid personality is not necessarily aware of any problem, and does not mind complying with compulsions and thoughts. While some make this distinction for diagnostic purposes, what interests me is the continuity.[30] The pathological form of obsession is OCD, particularly when it dominates the life of the person involved. But that same domination, when it is used to constructive ends, can be the root and bole of genius and creativity. As Rachman notes, "when people with creative energy succeed in putting their obsessional personality traits to constructive use, everyone benefits."[31]

In the requirement that the behaviors produce "marked distress" in the person, how one arrives at distress is crucial. The same behaviors in different cultures might produce different results. In other words, it takes a community, a culture, a family to make an obsessive. If your behavior, say the meticulous lining up of objects, is seen as an oddity, you will be distressed that you do it. If it is seen as the useful quality of a master bricklayer then you will not be distressed. In other words, "marked distress" is not a quality itself but rather a socially defined reaction. The other problem is that the neat distinction between the personality disorder (the person doesn't mind being obsessive) and the disorder (the person minds) is, even in the *DSM-IV* definition, confused by an acknowledgment that in some cases people "with OCD" won't be distressed by what they are doing or may even think that what they are doing is actually helpful or valuable. But in that case, they may be seen as having "poor insight."[32] Poor insight itself is a very socially dependent notion—if you agree you have the disorder, you have good insight; if you dispute this point or don't recognize yourself as having the disorder, then you might have poor insight.

One of the areas of concern to clinicians is that the cure rate for people with obsessive-compulsive disorders is not particularly good. In fact, one study notes that the group that fares the best is the one that is untreated, and generally outcome is unrelated to treatment.[33] More optimistic accounts, including ones with behavioral-cognitive therapy, can be found in the literature, but often they are based on assessments by the practitioner, which will always be more positive than a double-blind survey, which is largely impossible with this type of illness. With the advent of the use of drugs that affect serotonin levels in the brain like Prozac or Paxil, treatment outcomes have improved, although it is hard to say if this is really the case or just the result of the general optimism after the initial use of these drugs along with modified notions of cure and improvement. We will have to recall that drug choices in various epochs are tied to the viewpoints of those times. The widespread use of antianxiety drugs in the sixties proved useful to people with OCD, at least for a while, as did the use of antidepressants in the subsequent years. Psychosurgery, including lobotomy, was advocated for people with severe obsessional disorders, and that advice was discounted when psychosurgery went into decline as psychopharmacology picked up. Now that serotonin-increasing drugs, referred to as SSRIs (selective serotonin re-uptake inhibitors) have taken over the role of regnant chemical for affective disorders, we need to be aware of the epochal nature of such interventions. Also, new research using functional MRIs (fMRIs) and PET scans has produced data that may lead to new kinds of treatment.

The general point is that obsessive disorders are in some sense endemic, part of what it means to be human in the modern world. In Rachman and Hodgson's view, "Overall, it would appear that the outlook for obsessional patients is slightly worse than that for people suffering from other types of neurotic disorder."[34] Perhaps the attempt to cure OCD will be regarded by our successors as the equivalent to treating homosexuality or masturbation in the past—those pandemic diseases that proved so intractable to cure. Perhaps the current explanations—that the illness is dissociated from its times and that its victim is the object of a capricious set of brain activities or crossed wires or neurotransmitter imbalances—are not right.

METHOD FOR MADNESS

The methodological problem in this book is a considerable one. A researcher approaching the history of mental disorders, particularly those in the eighteenth and nineteenth centuries, is faced with a bewildering collection of pamphlets and books by a variety of practitioners. Unlike the study of literature, in which one author is very likely to have read the preceding body of novels or poems, and genuine tradition can be counted upon, in medicine, strangely enough, the approach is far less systematic. While certain doctors' works have great currency, say the work of Pinel, Charcot, or Freud, the majority of practitioners, even if they publish, are essentially unknown to each other. Only with the growth and development of professional medical organizations and their resulting journals and congresses do we begin to see the attempt of the medical profession to create and normalize diagnoses and treatments. Those organizations provide kinds of linearity, although such organizations also tend to reflect the whims, fancies, trends, and, yes, obsessions of their own times. Further, since the causes of and cures for mental illness are extremely uncertain and obscure, even in our own time, it is very difficult for any single practitioner to prove his or her approach correct. The history of the treatment of mental illnesses is a veritable sideshow, mountebank performance, and medicine show in which a raft of treatments floats through a sea of mental illnesses. The most respected practitioners have relied on and used the most astounding set of treatments imaginable from (literally) bromides of doubtful to pernicious value, from the use of hot or cold water baths, the use of restraints, electricity, heavy metals, hypnosis, purges, pain, poultices, bloodletting, irritants, fresh air, and on and on. Even with the current use of SSRIs, we have no assurance that the treatment is working, will continue to work, and is the final way of dealing with a condition. So there is no true unanimity, no solid ground, for a social and cultural research methodology into an area like obsession.

Then there is the problem of reliability and accuracy of sources. As with any history, the documents one deals with are themselves biased and of their time. Is there, then, a solid footing on which the medical historian can stand concerning a mental state and a set of diagnostic conditions? Is there a location of sanity and objectivity from whose heights one can survey the mad terrain? The answer is, not very likely. In addition, different camps will take differing positions on the nature of obsession, its definition, and the way in which the term can be applied. Psychologists will see the term one way, psychoanalysts another, cultural historians a different way. My hope is that this work will open a discussion about something that is all around us and for that reason appears somewhat mysterious, somewhat obvious, and completely blurred by its very proximity. As Marshall McLuhan once famously noted, "Whoever discovered water, it wasn't the fish." And so in this rediscovery of the obsession that is all around us, may we hope that we aren't exclusively of the finny breed.

I am well aware of the pitfalls of the genre of study I am about to engage in—the historical and cultural study of what is seen as a "new" phenomenon. Such a study has familiar contours. First is the model that relies on a strong sense of then and now—showing how things were different in the past and how by a certain date a new mode of thinking, acting, feeling, or doing had arisen. Second, in this genre the author argues for the invention of something new in culture and society and then goes on to show how that new thing then proliferated in the Western (or whatever) world. Finally, the author shows how important and all encompassing this phenomenon is and has been.

The pitfalls of this approach are obvious. Can one say that heterosexuality or sexuality or masturbation or fatigue or attention or scientific management of labor began on a particular date? To do so, one has to ignore to some extent or explain previous instantiations of what seem like sexuality or masturbation or whatever. Then one has to scour the literature for all occurrences of the new phenomenon. That task alone is herculean and necessarily arbitrary. How do we know that we have all the texts? Can one additional text change everything that one has assumed before? One has to make all kinds of categorical claims and disregard the sneaking evidence that might confound one's large claim. In writing my own history of obsession, I will of course enter into this genre, engage in some of these tactics, but I hope that by being aware of its pitfalls and limitations, I may be able to avoid the most egregious hazards of this kind of endeavor.

Nevertheless, the reader will be asked tentatively to go along with a set of assumptions that I have made. First and foremost is to accept the idea that while I am using the term "obsession" I could as easily have used "hysteria," "mania," "neurosis," or any of the other large categories of mental distress that have had various heydays in psychiatric discourse. I am drawn to the idea of obsession because it seems to characterize best the complexity of any medicalized way of thinking about the mind-body connection and a set of rules or norms supposed to apply to the way that the affects, thoughts, sentiments, and judgments are said to be interconnected. As I hope to show, the term "obsession" was applied to a loose set of behaviors that had been called various things at various times. The continuing interest, however, in obsessive behaviors has a complex set of instantiations and rebirths through the period from the eighteenth century to the present moment.

DISEASE ENTITIES

Therefore, a logical second assumption that I will ask readers to adopt is that both disease entities and treatments are very much products of the explanatory systems used and the times in which they arise. It might be controversial to assume that there aren't diseases as such but, rather, there are instead what have been called "disease entities." "Disease entities" might be the more complex way of describing the formerly discrete and unchallenged category of disease.[35] The concept of disease entities allows us to move away from the positivist kind of descriptive categories of disease and to think of diseases not as discrete objects but as ranges of bodily difference and reaction. To think about diseases in this way is not simply an intellectual fad.[36] The justification for this way of thinking is most particularly applicable to psychiatric disorders. In general medicine, or what might be called "classical" medicine, on which psychiatric medicine has tried to model itself, disease definitions often took their contours from somewhat consistent trends and manifestations of infectious diseases, which appeared to have relatively stable durations and symptoms, and a predictable set of outcomes.[37] Cholera, tetanus, influenza, plague, and so on can generally be put in fairly distinct taxonomic categories, and therefore they set the model for the modern scientific idea of disease, although there was a considerable body of medical literature around the idea of disease as a state, literally, of dis-ease, most readily translated as being out of sorts. That school of medicine considered the holistic, as we now say, state of health and therefore looked at disease as general rather than specific. Yet the dominant trend of European and American medicine came to focus on the life cycle, as it were, of specifically delimited infectious diseases caused by (later) identifiable bacteria or viruses.

But psychological disorders that include affective elements are quite another thing. Indeed, contemporary critics of psychiatry, many of whom were or are users of psychiatric services, have tried to call attention to the problematics of the medical model by refusing to call themselves "mental patients," preferring instead to use the term "mental health services users" or "consumers," and eschewing "mental illness" for the less medicalized "mental distress."[38] I will refer later to the way that medical doctors came to see obsession as within their purview. Another more provocative way of saying this is that doctors took over behaviors like obsession and came to see them as analogous to other "classical" diseases. As Michel Foucault even more provocatively noted of nineteenth-century practices, "psychiatry only has an imaginary relationship with scientific knowledge."[39] One might elaborate on what seems to be Foucault's mere denigration (although I believe he is using the notion of the imaginary in the Lacanian sense) in implying that the level of proof for nineteenth-century psychiatry cannot be equated with the level of proof in an ideal scientific experiment. The nineteenth century's notion of science would barely pass muster now, especially with notions of double-blind, randomized studies. In addition, psychiatrists were of course simply following along in a bourgeoning consumer culture that came to define being ill and going to the doctor as one more in a series of acts consumers might perform.

In saying this, let me caution again that I am not claiming that there are no diseases, that people with schizophrenia do not have a mental disorder, that people who are depressed are simply adopting a trendy mode of being in the early twenty-first century. I am, however, following along in the thinking of people like Ian Hacking, who explains very well the concept of what he calls "transient mental illness." Hacking notes that "mental illnesses," for example, fugue states, hysteria, anorexia, or attention deficit disorder, arise in society at given historical moments and then may as well disappear within twenty or thirty years. He notes that such illnesses are "real" but also notes their provisional status. And he highlights the feedback loops between diagnoses and diseases. The point is that we must consider that diseases, particularly ones as complexly envisioned as those we call mental illnesses, are distinctly tied to the historical moment, the set of expected behaviors and norms in society, and the paradigms of the observers and the observed. Juliet Mitchell, for example, notes the similarities between *saka,* a disease of the Taita people in Kenya, and hysteria, and claims that while hysteria is universal, it also changes through different historical periods and therefore "resists any such constraints or classification."[40]

I therefore assume the necessity for being aware of the way disease entities and corresponding explanatory systems arise in synchrony. Obsession is not a thing in itself. Indeed, one could argue that mental conditions can never be seen as discrete things apart from the nosological categories that form them. The cure system that helps define and change the mental or emotional condition is deeply linked to society in its broad and complex being, out of which the triggering behavior was selected.

A final assumption, and a fairly major one, that I will make in this book is that science, scientific medicine, and academic specialization—all of which achieve a kind of dominant formation in the nineteenth century in the Western world—are themselves not objective positions of knowledge but in fact aspects of the new problematics of obsession. This new method of knowledge requires all the hallmarks of obsessive behavior—fixation on one thing, repetitive interest in that thing, fixed attention to the details, copious notes, observations, repetitive and focused habits of study, and a strong compulsion to do all this. We can see in nineteenth-century literature a popular awareness that there is something strange and mad about science and scientists. Works like Mary Shelley's *Frankenstein,* Wilkie Collins's *Heart and Science,* Jules Verne's *20,000 Leagues under the Sea,* and Robert Louis Stevenson's *Dr. Jekyll and Mr. Hyde,* feature the visions of "mad scientists," driven to distraction by the obsessive nature of their work. Aware of this vision, the claim in this book is that science and by extension knowledge become, to some degree, the socially acceptable face of a culture of obsession, while the obsessive, the monomaniac, the neurasthenic, the sexual pervert, among others, become the extrojected object, selected for observation, by those engaged in the scientific study of obsessive behaviors.

In speaking this way, we need to consider a long and complicated approach to understanding a phenomenon like obsession, because in talking about categories of madness we are speaking of phenomena that have always been understood in different ways at different times. Even under the most favorable conditions we are talking about multiple states and shifting symptoms. Therefore, we have to posit a specific time and place where "obsession," as a shifting term, is understood one way, and then another specific time and place when it is understood another way. And so on through places and times. The result will not be, as is found in most psychiatric texts, that we arrive at the present, where we clearly understand what madness is and the past is all a confusing prolegomenon to a clear present and even clearer future. The truth probably is that madness remains as murky today as it has been in the past. Our contemporary paradigms and treatments are based on different kinds of measures and groupings than were used in the past, but we are by no means certain that the way we view things now is the way they actually will be twenty-five—let alone a hundred—years from now.

OBSESSING ABOUT LANGUAGE

The problem is further convoluted by the fact that the language we use to understand madness is itself a layered pentimento of concepts and terms that have arisen, been useful, become outmoded, and yet still persist. Since

the words we use will predetermine the object of study, we have to be careful that when we speak of obsession, or madness, or other like terms, we
understand that the objects so described through language may not correspond exactly to states of cognitive or emotional distress. Although we
are always looking at people, we describe what we see through words.

On a popular level, we talk comfortably about insanity, madness, and
mental illness as though each of those terms describes the same thing. We
feel capable of judging, at least informally, the level of sanity, neurosis, nervousness, or depression among our friends, family, and selves. Indeed, it
is family and friends who will often be the first to diagnose, suggest treatment, and also initiate legal action on behalf of a possible patient. Concepts of madness begin at home. Commonly, we can produce the phrases:
"I'm nervous." "He's crazy." "She's neurotic." "They're depressed." "He's
a lunatic." No one challenges us in ordinary life to define our terms, and
there is a community of opinion within a culture about human behavior
that sees all of these behaviors as part of something we have come to call,
again without much difficulty or thought, "mental illness." But, as we will
see, the exact discourse that should have jurisdiction over madness has
never been certain. The set of circumstances that allow a family member
to be concerned, seek professional help, and ultimately agree to have a
distressed relation brought in for assistance will always be based, circu-
itously, on the norms and expectations that have been developed mutually
over time by practitioners, patients, moralists, politicians, novelists, film-
makers, religious advisers, and so on.

Even our notion of being nervous is part of a long history of overlapping terms and explanations. When the various functions of the nervous
system were discovered from the eighteenth through the nineteenth century, people changed the way they spoke of their emotional states. Nerves
began to predominate and people began to think of themselves as "nervous" rather than "humorous." "Nervous energy," another term we still
use, was seen as a measurable way to discuss slack or tightened nerves.
When we say "my nerves were strained to the utmost" we mean that we
are "nervous wrecks." But the two meanings join only at the word itself.
Strained nerves relate to nerves as sinews, as John Milton, for example
meant when he wrote of Samson in 1646 that he was "straining all his
nerves" in pushing down the walls. The use of "nervous wrecks," in the
sense of an emotional disaster, like a shipwreck, began to be used at the
end of the nineteenth century. This comparison shows that when we now

use what we are thinking of as a relatively coherent linguistic system to explain our nervousness, we really aren't. What we see is an example of at least two overlapping meaning systems in regard to the body and the mind that we have come to use interchangeably through the persistence of language but the absence of sense.

When George Beard popularized the idea of neurasthenia in his 1881 book *American Nervousness,* he was taking advantage of the nerve as a location of energy and emotions. If your nerves were overly excited you were nervous; if your nerves were weak or exhausted (as in nervous exhaustion) you were neurasthenic. This model of medicine, in turn, was a product of a new way of seeing the body based on a model of balance in which too much or too little of something caused a disease, while the mean or norm was considered good health.[41] Every time we use the word "nervous" we signal the complex and confusing history of the body in relation to culture—the biocultural. So any discussion of obsession as a nervous disorder will reawaken many sleeping myths about the body and the mind.

OBSESSION VIEWED THROUGH TECHNOLOGY

At various historical moments, people had to ask of madness, Is this subject a medical one? A psychological one? A physiological one? A philosophical one? One of the points of this study is to trace the problematic of obsession as it moves through these different spheres of knowledge. It will be important to note the changes in the perception of obsession, as well as the perceivers of obsession, as both extend into different ways of knowing. Our current line of thinking is that all psychiatric states are a result of neurochemistry and brain activity. The general assumption is that "mind is what brain does."[42] So some clinicians and researchers who have miraculously persisted in reading my introduction up to this point will all the while have been shaking their heads at the ignorant insouciance of my project. They will tell you with certainty that it may be well and good to describe the social and cultural world surrounding disease, but that at core, at rock-hard base, is the reliable and now visualizable world of fMRI, PET, and various other imaging devices. They will tell you that they are on the verge of finding the place in the brain (the caudate nucleus of the basal ganglia or the cingulum or the prefrontal and orbitofrontal lobes) where OCD resides (see figs. 2 and 3). These images are intriguing, but their outcome isn't as certain as the scientists might claim. We are

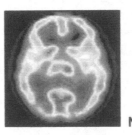

Normal Brain

FIGURE 2. Normal brain from *Archives of General Psychiatry* (copyright 1992–94 American Medical Association).

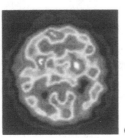

OCD Brain

FIGURE 3. OCD brain from *Archives of General Psychiatry* (copyright 1992–94 American Medical Association).

in the very early days of understanding the neurochemical and electrical activity of the brain. And, as a recent study has shown, simply providing images from fMRIs will increase acceptance among observers of even deliberately false and illogical explanations about brain function.[43] Technologies themselves will spawn new diagnoses[44] but in the long run we have seen that diagnoses may in fact change with further technologies. In other words, the seeming fixity and specificity of diseases can be buttressed by information provided by new technologies. But therefore, by definition, they can't be fixed or unchanging if they are dependent on a specific kind of technology, which itself can change or become obsolete.

A rather simple question that often gets lost in the very valid work being done in brain imaging and research into brain chemistry is, are the changes we are seeing a result of the disease or the cause of the disease? In other words, are people sad because they have low serotonin, or do people have low serotonin because they are sad? No one doubts that the brain changes and those changes can be measured, but is the OCD brain like that because the person is worrying and compulsive, or is the person obsessing and compulsive because of specific activities and chemistries independent of any individual will? This isn't merely a philosophical question but one with the utmost significance for this discussion of OCD.

In the end, many of psychiatry's assumptions are just assumptions. Mental distress is not easy to treat, nor can success rates be measured so easily. In looking at psychiatric disorders, we are not looking at an area of grand success. One study of OCD shows that without any treatment about a third of the patients get better, a third worse, and a third remained the same.[45] Chemical treatment of mental illness is currently the preferred mode, but we should not make the mistake of thinking that we have finally arrived at a solution through the psychopharmacological modality. Recent retrospective studies are casting serious doubts on the efficacy, safety, and utility of the recent fascination with SSRIs. Indeed, psychotherapists, behavioral therapists, psychoanalysts, and other researchers have made compelling arguments that talking cures and behavior modification can also create measurable changes in brain chemistry and electrical activity.[46] The history of mental distress in medicine shows us that there is a constant alternation among those who see madness as a larger intrapsychic experience, those who see it as a fundamentally physiological one, and those who see it as a combination of both. Of course, there is the additional perspective that comes and goes about the specific nature of distress—linking it to social and historical conditions. There is too the oscillating debate over whether drugs are the cure or whether talking and persuasion are the best methods to bring about a cessation of symptoms. Even talking cures are in debate at the moment, and there is much disagreement about whether psychotherapy should be a standardized practice based on scientific studies or whether it should be an intuitive and theoretical one.[47] While chemicals can and do affect the brain and behavior, the question remains whether mental illness is a chemical phenomenon, how well the chemicals work over a long haul, and how long-term use of and compliance in taking drugs will pan out. And of course, genetic arguments now abound as well.

But should obsession be considered a part of mental illness? That question is predicated on a notion that the thing we call mental illness is what it is—a medical phenomenon. Yet obsession seems both to partake of mental illness and to be separate from it. Indeed, there was a time when obsession was not considered an illness at all. In order to understand obsession, we will have to trace the development of obsession from where it begins as demonic possession and moves to a secularized fascination or curiosity and thence into obsession, the diseased state, and to do that, we have to look at the discourses surrounding obsession that would place it in a disease category.

I

Origins of Obsession

Obsession often involves a battle of selves in which a compulsive self struggles with an observing self. So it is apt that the earliest use of the word "obsession" has to do with war. In Latin *obsessio* and *possessio* were two aspects of besieging a city. *Possideo, -ere* and *obsideo, -ere* are two phases in the assault.[1] If you've obsessed a city, you've surrounded it, but the citadel remains intact; while if you possess the city, the walls have been breached and you've conquered the citadel and its citizens.

Given the battle metaphor, the term then came to be used in describing demonic possession. The devil is seen as the attacker and the victim as the city, with the citadel representing the soul. These terms were used in this sense since the third and fourth centuries, and the difference between possession and obsession seems to have been well understood at the time: the distinction was that in the case of *possession* the victim was unaware of the fact that she or he had been possessed by the devil because the devil had entered that person and had complete control over the soul. In the case of *obsession* that person was aware of being besieged by the devil since the demon did not have complete control, had not entered the city of the soul, and the victim could therefore attempt to resist.[2] The key for us in this discussion is that obsession means that the person is aware of the symptoms and possible cause of his or her behavior. This ability to know that certain behaviors are not controllable, but somehow are also not coming from within one's own desire or will, characterizes the disease of obsession.[3]

This linguistic usage will not change substantially until the middle of the nineteenth century, when we see the word being used in a distinctly psychiatric sense. Therefore, we will wait until that historical moment before pinpointing the emergence of obsession as a known category involving doing or thinking one thing too much, being aware of that activity, but being unable to stop it. For now, we will need to observe how the space was cleared for this concept of mental "illness."

How the religious explanation for obsessive behavior was displaced by a medical one involves a complex set of transformations. First, demonology had to be disconnected from physical maladies. Second, mental states had to be separated from physical states. Third, the nervous system had to be discovered. And fourth, a notion of partial insanity had to be developed that would allow for one to be "crazy" while at the same time being aware of being "crazy." This latter step would involve the democratization of madness, the turning of a kind of partial madness into a consumer object that would define, in a sense, what it meant to be human.

DEMONIC OBSESSION IN SHAKESPEARE

To follow the first step of the emergence of obsession, we need to see the course by which demonology was removed from the available explanatory system. For a good example of how Renaissance culture accepted the demonic possession/obsession model, we need look no further than Shakespeare's *Twelfth Night*. Malvolio is deemed a lunatic after he is tricked into believing that Olivia is in love with him. He is falsely and maliciously led to believe that she particularly wishes him to wear yellow stockings held up by cross-garters and to smile all the time as proof that he is in love with her. Naturally, his doing these ridiculous things causes Olivia, who is not in on the joke, to believe Malvolio is mad, as his enemies tell her. "He's coming, madam, but in very strange manner. He is sure possessed, madam." Sir Toby Belch says of Malvolio, "If all the devils of hell be drawn in little, and Legion himself possessed him, yet I'll speak to him." Of Malvolio, Maria says, "Lo, how hollow the fiend speaks within him." And Sir Toby advises Malvolio to "defy the devil. Consider he's an enemy to mankind." Later, when Malvolio is locked up in a dark room, the clown pretends to be a curate, Sir Topas, who has come to exorcise him.

Shakespeare could play on his audience's understanding that demonic possession was the cause of madness. The devil is seen as the cause of Malvolio's obsessive behavior, and the cure involves an act of renouncing the devil, prayer, and ultimately exorcism or divine intervention. The audience is also counted on to know that the gem topaz, which name the clown adopts in his false personality as a cleric, is a supposed cure for lunacy.[4] Here we might assume that most people in the audience would "know" that madness and possession were linked.

Of course, Malvolio isn't mad, really; he is only tricked into acting that way. But Lady Macbeth is perhaps closer to our notion of the obsessive than is Malvolio. Her madness might, in a post-Freudian era, be justly called obsessive-compulsive, with her delusions of blood and her need to wash constantly. While the doctor observes that her "heart is sorely charged," he emphasizes that what we are regarding is not a disease that a doctor can cure. "This disease is beyond my practice. . . ."

More needs she the divine than the physician.
God. God forgive us all. Look after her. (5.1.54, 69–70)

Obsession here is in the province of the clerical, and its treatment involves exorcism, not therapy. Indeed, major works on melancholy, for example, tended to be written by divines rather than physicians until the eighteenth century. So the demonic possession model continues.

DEMONS OUT; NERVES IN

The idea of the nonmedical, otherworldly origin of obsession seems to come to an end in the eighteenth century, and is signaled by a 1736 act of Parliament that abrogates all laws against "conjurations, inchantments, and witchcraft" that had been the grounds on which exorcism of the insane had been prosecuted.[5] The Protestants banned the idea of possession because the Catholic Church was seen as having the inside track on exorcisms, and banning the idea of possession was in effect a way of banning popery in general.

If you ban the idea that obsession means demonic possession, then you need another explanatory system. While demonic possession may have continued popularly into the eighteenth and nineteenth centuries, what ultimately replaced the system of demonic explanation was the nervous system. To illustrate the gap between these two explanatory modes let me present several incidents of what we would now call mass hysteria. Mass hysteria can be seen as group obsession in which people are driven to act, and can be aware of their actions, but are unable to stop.

On the February 15, 1787, a teenage girl working at a cotton factory in Hodder Bridge, Lancashire, decided to play a trick on her friend. She caught a mouse and dropped it down the other girl's dress. The girl with the mouse in her clothing "was immediately thrown into a fit" and remained so all that day and through the night.[6] On the following day, three more girls fell into similar fits and had violent convulsions that also lasted all day. Their symptoms were "anxiety, strangulation, and very strong convulsions; and these were so violent as to last, without any intermission, from a quarter of an hour to twenty-four hours, and to require four or five persons to prevent the patients from tearing their hair and dashing their heads against the floor or wall."

General concern began to mount as more and more girls, and one man, fell into varying states of confusion. Two days after the mouse-dropping incident, six more girls were seized with fits and convulsions. In this cotton factory of two to three hundred employees, work ground to a halt. Rumors began to spread that a disease had come from something in one of the bags of cotton that had been opened in the factory. By Sunday the eighteenth three more people fell into fits, and by the next day, eleven more.

The malady began to spread to other locales. Two of the newly stricken lived about two miles away, and three more worked at a factory about five miles away. These workers, and two more, were affected by the disease just from hearing about the epidemic. Now twenty-four workers were actively writhing in convulsions.

Dr. William St. Clare, a local physician from the nearby town of Preston with an interest in mental conditions, was summoned on Sunday the eighteenth. He arrived with a portable electrical machine.[7] Setting up his machine, which worked by manually cranking a generator, he began methodically shocking every patient. By this means, he stopped the epidemic. "The patients were universally relieved without exception." Once the workers "were assured that the complaint was merely nervous, easily cured, and not introduced by the cotton, no fresh person was affected."

This mass hysteria is noteworthy particularly for Dr. St. Clare's electrical apparatus. When cases like this occurred in earlier times, even just a bit earlier, the explanation was almost always attributed, again, to demonic possession. Indeed, eighty-six years earlier near Oxford, a group of children from the town of Blackthorn had been seized by attacks of "barking and howling like dogs . . . accompanied by violent rhythmic movements of the head and contortions of the face . . . when their breath failed they would one by one fall into a paroxysm like an epileptic fit."[8] Physicians were called then, as was Dr. St. Clare in the later story, but tellingly they could not stop the events. Demonic possession was the suspected cause, so medical doctors weren't of much use.

However, in a span of less than a hundred years, the new cause of the mass obsession in Lancashire was not the devil but "nerves." The solution to this problem was the "rational," if not accurate, application of electric shocks rather than any recourse to theological explanations or exorcisms. Both diagnosis and cure, handled by a physician, ended the epidemic. What then is the difference between the barking children and the convulsive factory workers?

Let me fast-forward another hundred years to introduce one more example of mass obsessive activity. In 1881 Sarah Bernhardt traveled to Moscow to perform *La dame aux camélias*. According to Gabriel Tarde, who heard about the event from a Russian doctor,

> In the fifth act, at the most dramatic moment, when the entire audience was so silent that you could have heard a pin drop, Marguerite Gautier [played by Bernhardt], dying of consumption, coughed. Immediately an epidemic of coughing filled the auditorium, and during several minutes, no one was able to hear the words of the great actress.[9]

Unlike the stories of barking children and fainting factory girls that appeared in newspapers as stories of general interest, the Bernhardt story is treated as a purely scientific observation from the very start. Tarde, the author of books on imitation and suggestion, simply uses the event to talk about the inherently "nervous" nature of this kind of group response.

Our Dr. St. Clare was able, at the end of the eighteenth century, to use the word "nerves" with some certainty in diagnosing the convulsing girls at the Lancashire cotton factory. Now, we use the term quite freely to specify a specific state of being, but the word is largely based on a presumption that nerves create nervousness or anxiety. That single word "nerves" actually marks a historical dividing line between seventeenth-century ideas of human behavior and eighteenth-century ones. The structure of nerves was discovered rather late in medical history, and the actual function of the nerves was certainly discovered even later. The first use of the term is linked not to the emotions but to the muscles—nerves were understood to be sinews, and to them were attributed strength. It wasn't until the eighteenth and then more generally the nineteenth century when they were thought to be the fibers of the emotions; then activity related to the emotions was linked to these parts of the body. Thomas Willis's book *Pathologiae cerebri, et nervosi generis specimen* (1687) introduced, by way of the English translator of his Latin work, the word "neurologie" as the "doctrine of the nerves." In the eighteenth century Dr. George Cheyne popularized the idea of a nervous disease, while his Scottish counterparts Robert Whytt and William Cullen furthered the idea of nerves. Whytt expanded the idea that nerves were responsible for a range of diseases, writing, "In my opinion the generality of morbid affections so depend on the nervous system, that almost every disease might be called nervous."[10] Cullen reinvented the term "neurosis." Assigning nerves a role in the emotions and energies was based on the charming bur erroneous assumption, at least initially, that nerves worked in the way that violin strings do— they vibrated sympathetically with each other. People were seen as having loose, tight, or aptly tuned nerves. Linked to this was some idea of humankind being connected on the emotional level—and thus the idea of human sympathy was seen as having a literal basis.[11] People whose nerves were too tight were seen as literally high-strung, nervously tense; those with too little tension were seen as weak-nerved, slack-willed, enervated.

Thomas Willis in the middle of the seventeenth century was the first to write a coherent account of the way nerves work in relation to the soul. It was he who coined the term "psycheology."[12] Abandoning humoral ideas, Willis came up with a more mechanistic approach to physiology that seems a kind of precursor to Locke's way of thinking about the brain. In Willis's system, the inner *spiritus animales* was stimulated by outer objects, thus creating sensations and therefore memory. Willis appropriated hysteria from an earlier tradition, but he broadened it away from the locus of the uterus to the nerves.[13] While it is quite common to laugh at "hysteria" as a strange and antiquated term, we would do better to understand that "hysteria," "spleen," "hypochondria," and "the vapors" were all ways of talking seriously about a particular kind of phenomenon in the history of mental and physical distress.[14]

CATEGORIES OF MADNESS

The laugh up the sleeve about previous mental categories should be balanced by a certain humility about our own fairly incoherent or perhaps arbitrary categories. It is therefore important that we try to understand the categories that precede the psychiatric diagnosis of obsession. Before the eighteenth century the categories of madness were limited to lunacy, melancholy, and idiocy, which are the oldest terms for mental illness in English. These latter were states that, while transitory, were also totalizing when they occurred. Lunacy was originally thought to have a periodicity related to the moon. A lunatic was someone who was insane, who raved, or who lost his or her wits. Melancholics were also called hypochondriacs, because the humor bile arose from the hypochondria, which we might call the area immediately below the diaphragm that included the liver, gallbladder, and spleen.[15] Melancholia, unlike the contemporary diagnosis of depression, was strongly equated with madness. Idiocy, which we would now consider to be unrelated to madness, was considered so because both madness and idiocy involved the loss of one's wits. What all these categories share, even lunacy, is that the definition, while periodic, is totally encompassing while it is occurring—one is completely lunatic, idiotic, or melancholic. George Cheyne called attention to this older view of madness when he wrote in the eighteenth century that "nervous distempers . . . are under some kind of disgrace and imputation, in the opinion of the vulgar and unlearned; they pass among the multitude for a lower degree of lunacy."[16]

The line drawn between melancholy and mania represented another way of thinking about the distinctions of madness. This major division is visually noted in the door over the entrance to Bethlehem Hospital which shows Caius Gabriel Cibber's twin figures of raving and melancholic madness. The maniac on the right is chained, while the languid figure on the left is the melancholic.

Thomas Arnold, writing in 1782, underlines this distinction in his book cataloging insanity:

Insanity, or madness, or lunacy, has usually been considered by medical writers, with some few exceptions, from the earliest ages, down to the present time, as consisting in two kinds; to one of which, they have almost unanimously given the name of Melancholy; and to the other that of Mania, Phrensy, or Fury.[17]

Of these, Arnold notes that both these states are "permanent."[18]

PARTIAL INSANITY

In the eighteenth century a new kind of mental distress became possible other than these two poles of permanent distress. This new form was characterized most clearly by its partial state; although periodic, when it was in place it did not disturb all the faculties of the mind. In essence such conditions were not totalizing in the way that lunacy and idiocy were. Rather these states presented a kind of middle ground in which one might be strongly affected by a mental problem but also clearly aware of the symptoms. Rather than "raving" or "furious," the person might be said to be able to articulate the conditions but powerless to resist. In effect, these states provided the deep background for the appearance of obsession as a modality, since obsession, as a disease entity, requires both an awareness of obsessive symptoms and an inability to stop the symptoms.

The group of diseases that had these partial qualities include hysteria (the female version),[19] hypochondria (the male), vapors, and spleen. While we are now somewhat unfamiliar with these conditions, in the eighteenth century they were well known, well distributed throughout the population, and well treated. For the sake of convenience, I have taken the liberty of calling these conditions collectively "the quartet." But there is more than convenience involved, since all of these conditions seep into each other diagnostically and taxonomically. George Cheyne called "the Hyp . . . a true Proteus" in that the symptoms of hypochondria were so variable.[20] They were characterized by bodily and mental states including what we now would call anxiety, depression, exhaustion, digestive problems, physical tics or manifestations, ennui, and so on. Cheyne's influential book *The English Malady* lists all of these states in its subtitle: *A Treatise of Nervous Diseases of All Kinds, as Spleen, Vapours, Lowness of Spirits, Hypochondriacal, and Hysterical Distempers, &c.*

With the advent of the quartet, the nature of madness changed. Now, no longer was the person totally taken up with the definition. One could be hysterical or have the vapors without that definition defining one completely. In addition, the quartet described a state that affected a rather large number of people, whereas madness encompassed a rather small number. This is the beginning of the opening up of the definitions of madness that, for any category short of severe mental illness, will ultimately include about a third of the population, according to Cheyne, with about half that number seeking treatment.[21] Subsequently, we will see the categories of neurasthenia, hysteria (again), neurosis, anxiety, and depression take over this overarching notion of what becomes a human condition. I will argue that while the older model of madness saw it as, according to one novelist, "the greatest misery with which our nature is afflicted,"[22] the newer model saw it as a badge of one's humanity. In this sense, the larger issue might be seen as the "democratization" of madness.

THE QUARTET

To understand this expansion of the category of madness from the restrictive sense of idiocy, lunacy, or melancholia to the larger and more capacious states around obsession, we need to follow along with the various components of the quartet. To begin with hysteria, by the eighteenth century the term began an expansion so that it no longer applied solely to women, although earlier theories had postulated the cause of the disease as being the strangulation of the uterus ("the suffocation of the mother" as it was called) or its rising and falling. William Harvey wrote in 1651 that "when the uterus either rises up or falls down, or is in any way put out of place or is seized with spasm—how dreadful then, are the mental aberrations, the delirium, the melancholy, the paroxysms of frenzy, as if the affected person were under the dominion of spells, and all arising from unnatural states of the uterus."[23] One notes that in the seventeenth century the idea of possession is still, vaguely, associated with hysteria in the idea that the person acts as if "under spells." But by the eighteenth century, physicians and nonphysicians had secularized this condition. Indeed, the public sphere became quite focused on hysteria, with many books appearing in print on this and other aspects of the quartet. These conditions became a subject of public discussion with a distinctly political and social dimension, unlike lunacy, melancholy, and idiocy. The point is that the treatment of hysteria and the manifestation of the diseases were not necessarily viewed as merely personal physiological or mental phenomena. Spleen and hysteria were seen as uniquely English diseases and were known collectively or severally as "The English Malady."

Cheyne attributes the disease to England particularly because of the "richness and heaviness of our food, the wealth and abundance of the inhabitants (from their universal trade), the inactivity and sedentary occupations of the better sort (among whom this evil mostly rages) and the humour of living in great, populous and consequently unhealthy towns."[24] For our purposes, hysteria, along with the vapors, melancholia, hypochondria, and the spleen—the quartet—were among the first elements of what would later be called "mental illness." The confluence of these states begin to create the elastic category of a new mental/physical/emotional being seen at once as pathological and paradoxically as normal.

These states, as we have seen, have a national character; sufferers were not at the bottom of the social scale, as was often the case with lunatics and idiots, but rather made up the cream of society. As Cheyne wrote, sufferers included those "of the liveliest and quickest natural parts, whose faculties are the brightest and most spiritual, whose genius is most keen and penetrating, and particularly where there is the most delicate sensation and taste both of pleasure and pain" not "fools, weak or stupid persons, heavy and dull souls . . ."[25] James Boswell took comfort in his symptoms, saying, "We hypochondriacks may console ourselves in the hour of gloomy distress, by thinking that our sufferings make us superior." Cheyne notes that people who are "tender" and who lead "sedentary lives, or indulge contemplative studies" are the most likely to suffer from "the passions."[26] Thus the sufferers of mental distress are often the richest, most sensitive, and most intellectual, as David Hume noted in 1734 when he described himself as ill with "the disease of the learned."[27] Cheyne goes into some detail: those who might indeed have the English Malady are "quick, prompt, and passionate . . . have a great degree of sensibility; are quick thinkers, feel pleasure or pain the most readily, and are of the most lively imagination."[28]

Because there had never been, up to this point, a distinct, articulated connection between medicine and madness—that is madness had not become mental illness or mental disease yet—there was no sense that doctors, particularly, should be involved in its treatment. Part of the reason that madness had not been seen as a disease was that with lunatics and idiots there could be only care, rarely, if ever, cure. In fact, it is amazing to realize that there were no doctors involved in German hospitals for the insane from the sixteenth through the eighteenth centuries. In England, physicians had been placed in charge of Bethlehem Hospital (or Bethlem, but better known as Bedlam) only at the end of the sixteenth century, but even then, for more than a hundred years thereafter, their role in the functioning of the hospital was minimal, not extending to more than a once-a-week visit. Even in that case, none of the physicians considered themselves specialists in insanity and none did any research into the treatment or the etiology of madness.[29] It was not until well into the nineteenth century that Bethlehem Hospital admitted medical students for clinical training.[30]

MELANCHOLIA

I have been arguing that madness changes its nature in the eighteenth century and moves from a totalizing state to a partial one, from a fairly exclusive state to a democratized one. That argument works fairly well, except for the case of melancholy. The melancholic was a figure well known before the eighteenth century. Depending on your sources, it is possible to trace the melancholic back to ancient Greece and Rome. As depression is defined now, a depressive is a person whose dejection is such that he or she may well be aware of it, like the obsessive who is able to comment on and be aware of his obsession. Yet despite awareness or insight, neither the melancholic nor the sufferers of vapors, spleen, hypochondria, and hysteria can effect a change by will. While obsession is seen as a disease of rationality and of will, melancholy is seen as a disposition or temperament. Both, again, are characteristic of intelligent people, scholars, writers, and in effect geniuses.

What is the difference, if any, between the melancholic and the sufferer from the quartet? We might want to begin with the observation that melancholia was not seen as a condition unique to medical treatment until the late eighteenth century when it more or less merged with the quartet. While some doctors involved themselves in the treatment of melancholia, notably, it was the divines who largely wrote treatises on melancholia. Bartholomaeus Anglicus, a thirteenth-century Parisian Minorite friar and professor of theology, articulated the Galenic principles of humors in *De proprietatibus rerum*. Yet he describes melancholy as something that includes what we would now call anxiety, paranoia, depression, and delusions. Sir Thomas More, who had been a Carthusian monk before he entered politics, wrote *A Dialogue of Comfort against Tribulation* (1553). The thirteenth-century Pope John XXI's work on madness was translated into English in 1550. The work included folk remedies "against madness," including roasting a mouse and dissecting and burning a frog. Andrew

Boorde, a physician but also a Carthusian monk and Bishop of Chichester, wrote on madness in 1552. Likewise, William Bullein was a divine and physician who advised in 1558 "good counsel" for the mad. Ludwig Lavater, divine of Zurich, wrote on melancholics in 1572. The famous *Anatomy of Melancholy* by Robert Burton was written not by a physician but again by an Anglican divine who became a madhouse keeper. As such his interest was primarily of a religious, not a medical, nature. Burton's vision is closer to the Galenic notion of a disease as an imbalance of humors affecting not particularly the brain but the entire organism's soul. Relief was ultimately in the hands of "the heavenly Physician." Both Timothy Rogers and Richard Baxter, who wrote books on melancholy, were also divines, the former a nonconformist minister and the latter the Bishop of Worcester.

In addition to being considered a religious issue, melancholia was not the rough equivalent to depression today. Saying so would be like equating black bile with a modern set of disease categories. When we think of depression now, we think of it in the terms of the democratization of madness. We believe that anyone can be depressed, know about it, and be rationally concerned about it. But if you look at the way that people wrote about depression before the eighteenth century, you can see that it actually is considered a condition that is the opposite of reason. Melancholy, like the rest of the so-called mental illnesses, has traveled a distance from the irrational disorder it was thought to be in the Middle Ages and Renaissance to the rational disorder it became later. For example, although the *DSM-IV TR* lists delusions as one feature of depressive episodes, that is not the defining character of mood disorders.

The melancholic is described by various sixteenth-century writers as fearful without reason, fearful of others without reason, laughing at sorrowful things, sorrowing over amusing things, talking too much or too little, having irrational delusions "such as they will break if touched" or that "because they hold the world in their hands they cannot open their hands," that they have no heads or they have asses' heads.[31] Similar delusions are noted by another writer of the era who says that melancholics persuade themselves they see or hear ghosts.[32] Melancholics can think of themselves as animals, earthen vessels, or divine prophets.[33] Reginald Scot in 1584 argued that people accused of witchcraft actually were not possessed by devils but were melancholics. His argument was based on the utter lack of reason displayed by such people. As he noted, "Melancholie abounding in their head, and ocupieng their braine, hath deprived or rather depraved their judgments, and all their senses."[34] They are so without reason that their disease cannot be understood as the kind of depression we now discuss. "For as some of these melancholike persons imagine, they are witches and by witchcraft can work wonders, and doo what they list: so doo other, troubled with this disease, imagine manie strange, incredible, and impossible things. . . . They imagine, that they can transforme their owne bodies, which never the less remaineth in the former shape . . ."[35] Indeed, Richard Baxter wrote in 1716 that melancholia was a "distemper" in which "the thinking faculty is diseased; and become like an inflamed eye, or a foot that is sprained or out of joynt, disabled for its proper work."[36] And Bernard Mandeville wrote in 1730 that "melancholy people . . . had as many several whimsies, and imagining themselves to be what they were not, stuck close to the absurdities of their fancies."[37] So unlike obsessive disorders, in which rationality remains functioning, melancholy was consistently seen in this period as an irrational disease. Moreover, diagnostic categories were not fixed, and melancholics were often simply called madmen.[38]

PHYSICIANS OR PHILOSOPHERS?

Unlike melancholia, which appeared incurable, disease entities like hysteria or spleen, with their wide application and shifting symptoms, were felt to be curable. Yet cure was not necessarily to be obtained from a physician. Thomas Arnold, a physician writing in 1782, explains that "medical people, therefore, being in a great measure excluded from this branch of practice, can have little or no valuable experiences of these [mental] disorders."[39] The reason for this exclusion is that madness requires the caregiver to have a place of confinement, and medical people generally did not have such places. Thus, "unhappy sufferers of this sort [are put] under the care of those persons, who, however ill qualified as to the knowledge of medicine, are furnished with the requisite conveniences for their government and safety."[40] A philosopher might have been just as likely to achieve results, since madness began to be defined philosophically as well as somatically. Indeed, Kant proposed that when a seemingly irrational criminal case is dealt with, "in this case the court cannot refer the question to the medical faculty but must refer it (because of its own incompetence) to the philosophy faculty."[41] In a poem written in 1809, Ann Bristow describes a "maniac" and appeals "to the metaphysician, the naturalist, or the skillful professor of anatomy," any of whom might be able to treat the madman.[42] J.-J. Belloc advised in the beginning of the nineteenth century that the medical profession foreswear any special expertise to make medical evaluations for the court, counseling instead that "the testimony of several neighbors or people who lived daily with this person or saw and conversed with him frequently" could do a better analysis of the person's sanity than any medical expert.[43] Another French physician wrote that "nothing would be more gratuitous than the presumption of a special capacity of physicians to evaluate mental competence in criminal cases." He added that any sane layman was "as competent as Monsieur Pinel or Monsieur Esquirol," the two most famous physicians of the age who treated the insane, since the layman has "the advantage of being foreign to all scientific prejudice."[44] On the other side of the debate, G. M. Burrows, a physician, argued strenuously against the notion that philosophers might be better at dealing with madness than doctors: "I strongly deprecate the impression, that none but philosophers can cure intellectual derangement."[45] Thus, it was with some difficulty and with a great deal of institutional foreplay that the medical profession managed to convince the world that madness was its special province and that the vagaries of the mind and perception were best called diseases and illnesses. As Andrew Scull notes, "Numerically, they [physicians] might still be a minority of those trafficking in madness, but their view of insanity as an illness was an increasingly influential one in upper-class circles."[46] Although there was no definitive physical or disease entity associated with madness, the notion that mad people or partially mad people were "ill" or "diseased" came to be seen as the proper explanation and physicians were seen as the logical practitioners. Indeed, Dr. Thomas Mayo, writing in 1817, noted that his purpose was "to vindicate the rights of [our] profession over insanity, and to elucidate its medical treatment."[47]

We will see that the takeover, as it were, of mental conditions by physicians was a crucial factor in the creation of the disease entity of obsession. The entrance of mental disease within bourgeois consumer culture through the expansion and infiltration of medical treatment into the home and domestic sphere was the first step in the creation of a category of mental illness which was demotic and widespread, which could affect a large number of people, which had both a national character and a mark of humanity associated with the assumption of the disease state.[48] Scull notes that medical men attempted "in thoroughly entrepreneurial ways to legitimize as authentic diseases new and milder (and presumably more treatable) varieties of 'nervous disorders'—the spleen, hypochondria, the vapors, hysteria—which apparently afflicted a more fashionable and desirable clientele than most of the Bedlam mad."[49] In order for this to happen, physicians had to be seen as the just and appropriate guardians of the mental health of the nation, and mental diseases had to be seen as following the arc of physical ones.

Paradoxically, the physicians' claim to be better at treating mental illness was based on the notion that the same treatments for the body in general would be salutary for the mind. General health would include mental health. The operative terms of "health," "illness," and "disease" would create the lexical environment to make the argument that the physician who best treats the body might best treat the mind. As John Conolly noted in 1830, it was crucial to make "medical men as familiar with disorders of the mind as with other disorders; and thus of rescuing lunatics from those whose interest it is to represent such maladies as more obscure, and more difficult to manage than they are."[50] Physicians could apply the same proven treatments to the mind as to the body and were better suited to do so than others. The paradox, however, is that a body-based approach to mental distress was becoming increasingly outmoded just as those very doctors of the body moved into the mind game. Dr. Francis Willis, the grandson of the man who treated King George, argued for physicians treating madness by decrying any notion that madness was a purely mental phenomenon. Medical treatment, he insisted was "the more necessary, because derangement has been considered by some to be merely and exclusively a mental disease, curable without the aid of medicine, by what are termed moral remedies; such as traveling and various kinds of amusements."[51]

HUMORS AND ORGANS

The most predominant eighteenth-century explanation, before the advent of a "nervous" etiology, for quartet states was the organ theory, in which specific organs were seen as dominating consciousness. Linked to this was a concept of humors and also of vapors. Humors interacted in creating an out-of-balance system; vapors arose from specific organs and affected other organs, particularly the brain. The vision of the body was as a kind of cauldron or vessel in which food and secretions created a composting inner world. We are used to laughing at Swift's *Mechanical Operation of the Spirit* and *Tale of a Tub,* but Swift's descriptions are actually very close to the medical theories of his time. If one compares Swift's explanation of madness as "a disturbance or transposition of the brain, by force of certain vapors issuing up from the lower faculties" and his notion of religious enthusiasts as being inspired by "wind" and "belching" with discussions of vapors rising up to the brain in the quartet, we will find similarities. Richard Blackmore's treatise on the spleen includes the following dramatic description:

> a depraved disposition of the stomach, and an impaired digestive faculty, accompanied with an eager desire to eat, and some hours after meals with great oppressions and grievous pain of the stomach; which likewise is sometimes so filled and distended with storms of hypochondriacal winds, that this receptacle, and the inferior neighbouring parts, seem a dark and troubled region of animal meteors and exhalations, where opposite steams and rarified juices contending for dominion, maintain continual war.[52]

The organ theory allows for one part of the system to affect the other, as when vapors rise from the stomach to the brain. This theory was not, I want to keep stressing, subscribed to only by crackpots and eccentrics. Even someone as practical as Boswell uses it to describe Dr. Johnson's symptoms. Boswell notes that when some "have fancied themselves to be deprived of the use of their limbs, some to labour under acute diseases, others to be in extreme poverty . . . when the vapors were dispelled, they were convinced of their delusions."[53]

THE DISEASE OF RATIONALITY

It is by no means clear that large numbers of people accepted a physiological, body-oriented notion of illness even in the eighteenth century. According to William Battie, one of the Enlightenment's theoreticians of madness, the source of insanity was precisely not physical but was rather caused by a "deluded imagination, which is not only an indisputable but an essential character of madness."[54] No mention is made of a physical component, since Battie stresses the imagination alone. Alexander Anderson at the end of the eighteenth century in the United States writes along the same lines, "Madness may be defined as a false perception of objects, depending on morbid sensation, with a belief in the truth of the suggestions of the senses, and in consequence of this, extraordinary and irregular efforts to atone some imaginary good or avoid some evil."[55] In this notion, madness is an error of perception, a false way of reasoning, a detour in the Lockean imprinting of sensations on the mind. Madness is a disease of rationality, and rationality is a human trait. Perhaps it is not uncoincidental that the mind should come to the fore at this time. John Locke, along with Hume and Kant, had begun to develop influential theories concerning the mind. As Locke himself noted

> The defect in Naturals [people with cognitive impairments] seems to proceed from want of quickness, activity, and motion, in the intellectual faculties, whereby they are deprived of reason: whereas mad men, on the other side, seem to suffer by the other extreme. For they do not appear to me to have lost the faculty of reasoning: but having joined together some ideas very wrongly, they mistake them for truths; and they err, as men do, that argue right from wrong principles.[56]

Madness is a form of incorrect thinking. Thus, ironically, madness becomes an emblem of being human and a reminder that we cannot always be rational. As Battie wrote of madness, we can "precisely discriminate this from all other animal disorders: or that man and man alone is properly mad."[57]

DEMOCRATIZATION OF MADNESS

What I am trying to describe is a movement to extend madness from a small number of people to a rather large number.[58] In so doing, the severity of the disease is moderated, a trendy medical aspect is put in the mix, and a social and intellectual cachet is added. The best and the brightest now are the target group for what is called mental illness. Madness becomes fashionable, national, and almost a requirement to be in the intellectual and social elite. By extension, even the nonelite wants this right. This kind of madness is related not only to national character but to the national economy as well. Cheyne refers to the financial disaster of what was called the "South Sea Bubble," in which many investors lost their money in a stock crash in 1720, saying "the S. S. & other disappointments & passions of the mind" had provided him with business and patients, owing to their mental and physical distress on losing their money. And this economic strain provided the key to the book written by physician John Midriff in 1721 called *Observations of the Spleen and Vapours: Containing Remarkable Cases of Persons of Both Sexes, and All Ranks, from the Aspiring Director to the Humble Bubbler,*

Who Have Been Miserably Afflicted with Those Melancholy Disorders since the Fall of South Sea and Other Public Stock. Another writer noted in *Applebee's Journal* of January 1721, "We are assured, that the number of distemper'd heads is so strangely encreas'd for some months past, by the sudden rising and falling of men's fortunes and families, under the operation of South Sea vomits . . . that there is not room to be had among the private Bedlams or mad-houses as they are call'd, throughout the town."[59]

This extension of madness, seen as a product of economic stress, is almost universal and can be seen as the equivalent of the extension of the political franchise occurring at the same time. Capitalism and the material woes associated with the development of markets are even now seen as a great contributor to well being. With the expansion of the middle classes, we see that financial worries, particularly based around the volatility of markets, variations in supply and demand, the rise and fall of stocks all contribute to mental conditions.[60] Madness, as it transforms into the new "mental illness," is distributed throughout the population, since, for example, almost everyone has financial problems. Madness, in the old sense, is singular and rare; mental illness, in the new sense, is plural and common. In that manner, it is as democratic as death and taxes.

OBSESSION AND GENIUS

This expansion of the category of madness is aided by discussions of the tenuous line between madness and genius. Alexander Anderson in 1796 allows for a continuum between madness and genius, writing "that we can scarcely say where rationality ends and folly begins. No less difficult would the task be to determine the point at which madness commences, since very inordinate indulgence of the passions partakes of it, and even low spirits and absence of mind may be reckoned as slighter degrees of the same affection."[61] He goes on to acknowledge that great genius is itself like madness, and both Christ and St. Paul were accused of being "demoniac, or in other words a madman." Echoing Plato, he continues: "The transition from poetic ardor to madness is easy; hence some of the most sublime of imagination have been the productions of a disordered mind."[62] Samuel Tissot writes that "the brain of Blaise Paschal was so vitiated by passing his life in the laborious exercises of study, thought, and imagination, that certain fibres, agitated by incessant motion, made him perpetually feel a sensation, which seem'd to be excited by a globe of fire being plac'd on one side of him;

and his reason being overpower'd by the disorder of his nerves, he could scarce banish the idea of the fiery glove being actually present."[63] Thomas Arnold writes in 1782 that "it has been commonly asserted, that persons of great abilities, and genius, are more liable to madness than men of inferior understandings. . . . It is true, that persons of great inventive genius, of fine imagination, and of lively feelings, if not blessed with great judgment, as well as with the best moral dispositions, are so situated upon the very verge of madness, that they easily fall into it."[64] This thought is carried on in 1807 when Thomas Trotter observes of studious men that "the mind itself, by pursing one train of thought, and poring too long over the same subject, becomes torpid to external agents. . . . Hence the numerous instances of dyspepsia, hypochondriasis and melancholia, in the literary character."[65]

This expanded cultural view of mental illness is significant. Indeed, culture and society became fascinated with this new form of madness. A survey of medical writing in the eighteenth century in England, Europe, and Russia shows that publications on madness and the malfunctioning imagination far outnumbered all others.[66] The sales of books written by doctors and others about insanity, melancholia, the quartet, and other states of mind were considerable. In fact, William Perfect's 1787 book *Select Cases in the Different Species of Insanity, Lunacy, or Madness,* the first publication of psychiatric case materials, went through seven editions, making it one of the best-selling books on the subject, exceeded in editions only by Burton's *Anatomy of Melancholy.*[67]

PARTIAL INSANITY AND THE LAW

Much of this writing was taken up with arguments about the nature of insanity and the possibility for its cure. Once one allows that insanity is not a permanent condition but can be cured, a notion of intermittency, partiality, and continuum appears. When that is the case, the law, particularly the legal defense by reason of insanity, comes into play. Before the eighteenth century, the notion that one had to be completely mad to be exonerated from criminal responsibility obtained. Since the twelfth century when Henry de Bracton articulated in English law the notion that a "total lack of discretion and understanding" was the key to an insanity defense, the regnant concept was that the defendant had to be of a totally "unsound mind."[68] This concepts continues so that "only absolute madness, absolute deprivation of memory, could define the 'furious man.'"[69]

In the eighteenth century we can see the transition from absolute to partial madness. If we look at a celebrated trial of 1723 in which a Mr. Arnold was brought before the court for his part in a plot to kill the king, we see Mr. Justice Tracy addressing the jury and pointing out that for acquittal "it must be a man that is totally deprived of his understanding and memory, and doth not know what he is doing, no more than an infant, than a brute or a wild beast."[70] This absolute standard changed radically by 1760 at the trial of Earl Ferrers. The defense was "occasional insanity of the mind," in which Ferrers testifies that "at the time of this action, I could not know what I was about."[71] Dr. John Monro, physician superintendent of Bethlem, testified at these proceedings in what seems to have been the first recorded instance of an expert "psychiatric" witness in a criminal trial. He noted that temporary total insanity was an acceptable defense. Yet ultimately that defense did not prevail in this trial, partly because Ferrers, who was deprived of legal counsel and had to defend himself, paradoxically tried to show with his own wits that he was out of his wits at the time of the murder. Perhaps because of that tactic, Ferrers was convicted and executed. In 1800, the Hadfield decision introduced the concept of delusion. James Hadfield, a war veteran with considerable brain damage, made an attempt on the life of George III. Thomas Erskine undertook Hadfield's defense and made a sweeping conclusion about insanity, saying, "Delusion, therefore, where there is no frenzy or raving madness, is the true character of insanity."[72] This qualification changes the very nature of insanity and tilts it toward the notion that "true" insanity is embodied in the person who can think rationally and speak rationally, but who has some particular embedded delusion. As Joel Peter Eigen notes, "An act could be coolly and 'rationally' planned, yet still be the product of a madman, owing to his delusive construction of the circumstances surrounding the event."[73] This ruling in Hadfield's favor and others like it paved the way for a category of mental illness primarily characterized by delusion, obsession, compulsion—all of which imply a level of rationality coexisting with a level of irrationality.

OBSESSIVE AS GOOD CITIZEN AND CONSUMER

My goal here has been to describe with archival material a slow shift that opens up both a category of illness—mental illness—and a particular type of mental illness based around obsessive thinking and compulsive activities. In other words, I'm trying retrospectively to see how a space opens in a cultural field. One could easily object that what I am doing is based on a fallacy of trying to find in the past structures for things that don't yet exist. In other words, I'm engaging in a kind of retrospective fallacy. I grant that this is entirely possible. On the other hand, there is, I think I've shown, sufficient historical and archival evidence that a major shift occurs in the eighteenth century from a view of madness as a totalizing phenomenon afflicting a few poor souls to one that is seen as endemic to the culture, and one that is no longer totalizing to the individual, but rather partial and affecting only one part of the mental apparatus. This development allows for obsessions and compulsions to move to the fore, to signify a very human essence, and to be a characteristic of genius, good birth, and good character. In other words, obsession now becomes the prime example of mental "illness" for much of the nineteenth and twentieth centuries. Obsession becomes both the symptom and the cause of mental disease. It becomes the method by which disease is observed, and the disease itself. In addition, it becomes something the culture at large both wants and fears.

One sees in works and authors of the latter eighteenth-century representations of an increasingly complex kind of madness such as I have been describing. Indeed, to be an author, a thinker, or an intellectual during this time seems to have required mental symptoms found in the quartet. This situation might be paralleled in modern life by the necessity of having a "neurosis" and being in therapy, as Woody Allen might insist. For example, Samuel Richardson was a hypochondriac, according to his physician friend George Cheyne, the author of *The English Malady,* who wrote to Richardson, "You are a true genuine Hyppo now with all its plainest symptoms."[74] Isaac Newton, along with James Boswell, Samuel Johnson, and many others were too. The eighteenth century saw the rise of what was called "sensibility" or "sentimentality." This new interest in affective life was a complex cultural reaction. Implied in "sentimentality" was the need to respond to characters, situations, and writing in general, both as author and reader, with a heightened emotional distress. The consequence of this kind of sentimentality was a special interest in these emotions in psychological settings. As Raymond Stephanson emphasizes, "The symptoms of nervous disorder or weak nerves (tears, physical agitation, fainting, etc.) now became important evidence of moral and social virtues."[75] Indeed, by 1771, when Henry Mackenzie published the signal novel for this era, his

The Man of Feeling, one could, indeed should, have a male protagonist cry virtually incessantly. A cult of reading works that made one cry and feel sentimental emerged in this period, as a bookseller in another novel suggests when he declares that a "crying volume . . . brings me more money in six months than a heavy merry thing will in six years."[76]

A certain cachet developed, a notion of being fashionable, in having one of these partial, intermittent conditions. Recall that rather than the stigma of lunacy, the quartet heralded the honor of being a proud citizen of a nation known for "the English Malady." One writer refers in 1725 to the vapors as "a modish disease."[77] Cheyne and others, as has been noted, emphasized that the malady came from an advanced state of living, of urban civilization. And the modishness of Bath, along with increasing "scientific proof" of the efficacy and composition of spa waters,[78] arose in the eighteenth century in conjunction with this new ideology of consumer-oriented, partial and curable disease states. Indeed, the Bath General Hospital was established in 1741 to provide scientific proof that the waters at Bath were efficacious so that the wealthy clientele would have more reason to go to Bath rather than rival spa locations.[79] This new consumerist insanity held true not only for England but for France as well, with writers like Rousseau and Tissot contrasting the clear, grounded sanity of the peasantry living the older, stable life, in comparison with the more civilized but more rushed and hectic form of life provided by the city, which encouraged these nervous maladies. Thomas Arnold, too, notes that "among the poorer and less civilized inhabitants of modern Europe, we hear but little of this [mental] disorder."[80] And Thomas Trotter echoes all these theorists, noting that "the uncivilized being is free from all those mental disquietudes, as well as bodily ailments" of civilized beings.[81] Rousseau's noble savage is, by definition, sane, but Rousseau and other denizens of the city and the academy might well be insane.

WE'RE ALL NERVOUS

Indeed, the modishness of the quartet easily shifted to the modishness of nervous diseases. One physician who wrote about the invalid trade in Bath noted in 1786 that before Whytt's treatise on nerves came out, "people of fashion had not the least idea that they had nerves," but after that, "the term [nerves] became fashionable, and spleen, vapours, and hyp [*sic*], were forgotten."[82] Cullen invented the term "neuroses" to distill all the nervous diseases into one category. As he wrote:

> In a certain view, almost the whole of the diseases of the human body might be called nervous: but there would be no use for such a general appellation; and, on the other hand, it seems improper to limit the term, in the loose inaccurate manner in which it has hitherto been applied, to hysteric and hypochondriacal disorders, which are themselves hardly to be defined with sufficient precision. In this place I propose to comprehend, under the title of neuroses, all those preternatural affections of sense and motion.[83]

This new era in which almost all maladies might be thought of as nervous further expands the reach and grasp of the medical profession into the realm of the new "nervous diseases" while it ramps up the connection between the mind and the body as well. George Cheyne wrote that "all nervous distempers whatsoever from yawning and stretching, up to a mortal fit of an apoplexy, seem to me to be but one continued disorder . . . [in] the nerves in particular."[84] The modality of obsession emerges from this new synthesis and expansion. It now seems clear that we have moved from demonic possession, to humoral/organ theory, and finally to the matrix of the nervous system. The nerves are the physical link to the mental—they are dissectible, discernable, and physical, yet their effects are metaphysical, symbolic, and affective.

Contemporary literature provides a window into this transition. For example, *The Man of Feeling* not only embodies male hysteria and hypochondria in its main character Harley and his lachrymose sensibility but also tellingly includes a visit to Bedlam, making explicit the connection between the virtues of sentimentality and obsession and the dangers of insanity. The inmates of Bedlam are by definition incurables, presenting us with the older view of insanity as totalizing and permanent—a "distress which the humane must see, with the painful reflection, that it is not in their power to alleviate it."[85] Some of the inmates are chained, violent to themselves and others, but a different area houses ones who are not dangerous. All of this group whom Harley and friends meet are people from the upper classes—of the upper bourgeoisie, gentry, and nobility. The fact that this slice of society has become mad illustrates the notion that madness comes from extreme sensibility and intelligence. The inmates display various kinds of obsessions. One is a mathematician who "fell a sacrifice. . . . to the theory of comets" and who is disappointed by a deviation in his calculations; another is businessman who lost all his money on the stock market. A third is a famous schoolmaster who was obsessed with determining the correct pronunciation of Greek verbs. Harley's guide himself turns out to be deluded, believing himself to be the Chan of Tartary; finally there is a noblewoman whose heart was broken in love. All of these people are consistently mad, showing us that the older model still applies to lunatics, but the fact that their madness is caused by focusing too closely on a single subject, in effect obsessing, rather than by somatic causes—the quartet, organs, or humors—tells us that we are looking at the adoption of a newer model.

It is worth considering the extent to which the modishness of partial insanity caught on through the act of reading. Too much study and too much reading can lead to obsessive disorders. Novels like *The Man of Feeling* may portray this new madness, but the act of novel reading also causes it. Just as Don Quixote became deluded through reading about the feats of knights, modern Quixotes did so as well—but now rather than a popular notion of madness there was a scientific explanation. This is given by Thomas Trotter, among others, who asserts that "novel reading . . . is one of the great causes of nervous disorders."[86]

CALEB WILLIAMS: THE FIRST OBSESSIVE NOVEL

In William Godwin's strange book *Caleb Williams,* published in 1794, an intermittent madness centering on obsessions of various kinds is central to the novel. This work merits some closer scrutiny because it is probably one of the first literary productions to focus in detail on this new incarnation of obsession, without actually using that term. Anyone who has read *Caleb Williams* becomes immediately aware that it is a strange book for the eighteenth century. Its strangeness comes, it seems, from its dwelling on characters that are "modern" in the sense of being mentally disordered, and particularly with a kind of mental disorder we might call obsessive. One can of course point to earlier instances of obsession, notably Uncle Toby's hobbyhorse in *Tristram Shandy* or Lovelace's erotic focus in *Clarissa.* But those characters are not the main protagonists. Neither do they seem aware of their obsession, and in that sense have not fully conformed to the self-aware aspect of obsession. Additionally, Lovelace's obsession for Clarissa fits into the long list of men with erotomania that characterizes Jacobean and Restoration comedies. In neither case are lovers thought to be seriously mad, although they may seem to be mad in silly, or funny, or dangerous ways. But in *Caleb Williams* we see obsession as a deep and serious problem that makes people clinically insane in the ways that we have been discussing. The nineteenth century looked back at Godwin's novel and saw it as illustrating monomania.[87] And it is with the category of monomania that we get the first birth pangs of the actual use of the term "obsession."[88]

The main villain, Mr. Falkland, is described throughout the novel as subject to melancholy, but he also has moments of greater or more intense madness. As Caleb notes, "There was a solemn sadness in his manner. . . . These symptoms are uninterrupted, except at certain times when his sufferings become intolerable, and he displays the marks of a furious insanity. At those times his language is fearful and mysterious, and he seems to figure to himself by turns every sort of persecution and alarm."[89] During Falkland's "frenzy," described as "symptoms," he would "strike his forehead, his brows became knit, his features distorted, and his teeth ground one against the other" (9). Falkland's paroxysms eventually take the form of an obsessive vendetta against Caleb.

Interestingly, Caleb describes himself as consumed by "curiosity," which he admits is "my ruling passion" (124). This ruling passion begins to look like what will shortly be called monomania or idée fixe. Indeed, this curiosity looks a lot like a kind of obsession, or what we now call "ruminative" thinking. As Caleb notes,

> Curiosity is a principle that carries its pleasures, as well as its pains, along with it. The mind is urged by a perpetual stimulus; it seems as if it were continually approaching to the end of its race; and as the insatiable desire of satisfaction is its principle of conduct, so it promises itself in that satisfaction an unknown gratification which seems as if it were capable of fully compensating any injuries that may be suffered in the career. (128)

But as with ruminative thinking that continues, promising an end without producing it, Caleb points out how in Falkland's curious obsessing "there was no consolation" (128).

This obsessive curiosity belongs not simply to Caleb or Falkland, but to both. It is the thing that links them in their *folie à deux* and makes them doppelgangers in some sense.

On Caleb's side, the curiosity involves the character and motivation of people, a trait that first launched him into this plot by his discovery of Falkland's secret of homicide. This attentiveness, or as Caleb puts it, "the constant state of vigilance and suspicion in which my mind was retained" allows him to pay particular attention to "what passed in the mind of one man, and the variety of conjectures into which I was led, appeared as it were to render me a competent adept in the different modes in which the human intellect displays its secret workings" (129). What we see in development here is two-fold: Caleb is, through his obsessive attention to human behavior, a kind of analyst of the psyche. He is also an incipient detective, and indeed, this novel is one of the first forerunners of the genre of detective fiction.[90] The desire to create a story with a secret that must be solved by the narrator and the reader, and in which both must pay careful attention to trivial details and a range of human behavior, creates a kind of literary work that will become familiar in the nineteenth and twentieth centuries. But we could equally say that the activity of reading and writing such a novel requires a kind of obsessive attention that would later be translated into the more detailed behavior of the alienist or analyst. Caleb's curiosity on this score allows him to become an analyst or detective and so to "watch him [Falkland] without remission. I will trace all the mazes of his thought."[91]

The increasing psychological attention of novels parallels the growing interest in mental life. We tend to think of the psychological novel as coming from a philosophical tradition with writers like Locke and Kant, but for the reading public, the attention to the "mazes" of thought may well have come from a much larger transformation of the biocultural public sphere of which Locke may have been only one aspect. The development of interest in a physiology of the mind, of popular explanations for mental and emotional states, may have been a significant motor for this kind of cultural interest and transformation. Caleb's role as analyst of others and himself could only have been interesting to a culture already preoccupied with the inner states of people. Indeed, Caleb blames himself for his analysis, saying, "Why should my reflections perpetually centre upon myself?—self, an overweening regard to which has been the source of my errors!" (336). Yet the focus on the self, the obsession with a haunting aspect of the self or other, seems to be a new cultural development, linked as it was to a popular consumption of a new way of seeing insanity.

Godwin links curiosity with this new type of intermittent or partial madness, saying, "Curiosity is a restless propensity and often does but hurry us forward the more irresistibly, the greater is the danger that attends its indulgence" (118). As Barbara Benedict notes of Caleb, he no "longer possesses curiosity; it, as an irrational impulse, possesses him."[92] Indeed, we might see this way of putting things as characteristic of the new mental "illness," which seizes on the rational faculties and makes them hyperrational, as it were.

Caleb connects the law with partial madness, first promulgated in the Ferrers trial of 1760, by saying of Falkland that "his fits of insanity—for such I must denominate them for want of a distinct appellation, though it is possible they might not fall under the definition that either the faculty or the court of chancery appropriate to the term—became stronger and more durable than ever."[93] To emphasize, however, that this state of mind or disposition that he is describing in Falkland is not like the insanity the court has previously upheld—complete, total, and all encompassing, Caleb warns,

> The reader however must not imagine, though I have employed the word insanity in describing Mr. Falkland's symptoms, that he was by any means reckoned for a madman by the generality of those who had occasion to observe him. It is true that his behaviour at certain times was singular and unaccountable; but then at other times there was in it so much dignity, regularity and economy, he knew so well how to command and make himself respect; his actions and carriage were so condescending, considerate and benevolent, that far from having forfeited the esteem of the unfortunate or the many, they were loud and earnest in his praises. (132)

Falkland's insanity is precisely a type that allows for a sane person to have a particular focused insanity—to be obsessed in the newer sense of partial and even self-aware.

Likewise, Caleb's own behavior fits this description as well. When Caleb becomes convinced that Falkland is a murderer, he decides impulsively to open a forbidden trunk containing incriminating evidence during the distraction offered by a fire in Falkland's mansion. As Caleb says, "My act was in some sort an act of insanity. . . . It was an instantaneous impulse, a short-lived and passing alienation of mind." He points out that the fire in the house caused a sympathetic change within him so that "by contagion [I] became alike desperate" (139).

Perhaps following the lead of his daughter Mary Shelley when she wrote *Frankenstein,* Godwin included an appendix in a later edition about what it was like to write his novel. This completely new interest in the mental state of the author at the time of composition signals the growing interest in obsessive activities like novel writing, in the workings of the mind, and we might say the temporary delusion of novel reading and writing. Godwin's description is full of anxiety as to the success of the work. He pinpoints the area in which "my imagination reveled the most freely," which he describes as "the analysis of the private and internal operations of the mind, employing my metaphysical dissecting knife in tracing and laying bare the involutions of motive, and recording the gradually accumulating impulses" of his characters (351). Godwin sees himself as a surgeon operating on the nervous system—a move that parallels the growing interest in neurology and psychiatry that we are tracing.

DR. JOHNSON: A CASE HISTORY

Another author who lived at the end of the eighteenth century—Dr. Samuel Johnson—is a good example of someone who illustrates the point that the quartet is a general expansion of madness without the totalizing effect of being mad. Boswell, who published his biography of Johnson in 1791, had to defend Johnson against the claim that he was mad. Retrospectively, Johnson has been assumed to have Tourette syndrome, which may account for his oddities as well as his accomplishments.[94] In any case, when we look at Boswell's comments in the light of this discussion, we see immediately that Boswell and Johnson found themselves in the middle of this changeover in the nature of madness. Johnson referred to himself as "mad" on various occasions, living in dread of losing his reason. Boswell, as a younger man who came of age, as it were, in the elaboration of the quartet, and himself an acknowledged "Hyp," argues for a different view of madness. Boswell points out this difference in views: "I am aware that he himself [Johnson] was too ready to call such a complaint by the name of madness. . . . But there is surely a clear distinction between a disorder which affects only the imagination and spirit, while the judgment is sound, and a disorder by which the judgment itself is impaired."[95] The distinction is initially made between a totalizing view and a partial, temporary, or intermittent view. "This distinction," Boswell notes, "was made to me by the late Professor Gaubius, of Leyden . . . and he expounded thus. 'If (said he) a man tells me that he is grievously disturbed, for that he imagines he sees a ruffian coming against him with a drawn sword, though at the same time he is conscious it is a delusion, I pronounce him to have a disordered imagination; but if a man tells me that he sees this, and in consternation calls to me to look at it, I pronounce him to be mad.'"

Boswell names the "morbid melancholy" which "afflict[ed] him [Johnson] in a dreadful manner" and "overwhelmed" him with "hypochondria . . . perpetual irritation, fretfulness, and impatience . . . dejection, gloom, and despair, which made existence misery" (1:23). He adds that "from this dismal malady he never afterward was perfectly relieved; and all his labours, and all his enjoyments, were but temporary interruptions of its baleful influence" (1:23). We can see here a puzzle over the definition of madness—is it totalizing or is it intermittent? How can one be reasonable, indeed a genius, and "at the same time visited with a disorder so afflictive?" (1:24). Clearly aware of the current discussion about madness, Boswell notes that "Johnson was an HYPOCHONDRIAC, was subject to what the learned, philosophical, and pious Dr. Cheyne has so well treated under the title of 'The English Malady'" (1:24). Boswell takes pains to point out the notion of the intermittent nature of the illness, as he writes, "The powers of his great mind might be troubled, and their full exercise suspended at times; but the mind itself was ever entire" (1:24). Boswell concludes that it is obvious that Johnson thought himself mad and "insanity . . . was the object of his most dismal apprehension," but just because "his own diseased imagination should have so far deceived him," was no reason that "his friends should have given credit to his groundless opinion" (1:25).

We can see in Samuel Johnson a change taking place in the construction of madness and an expansion of the franchise on being mad. I use the word "franchise" deliberately because there is something democratic in the notion that each person can become mad. Obsession is now no longer demonic, but has become a demotic form of madness that anyone can acquire. If each propertied man in the eighteenth century, and I use those descriptors advisedly, has a right to vote, each one also has a right to be splenetic, vaporous, hysterical, or hypochondriacal. Indeed, as we have seen, there is a certain cachet in being mentally affected. We begin to see a trend in the promotion of obsession as a trait that confers a complexity, an implication of genius, on the possessor. At this point, we can see that Boswell, while privately proclaiming himself distinguished by hypochondria, argues publicly for Johnson that his affliction is both medically sound and noninvasive of Johnson's creative and reasoning faculties.

It is interesting to note that about fifty years later, Thomas Babington Macaulay's *Life of Samuel Johnson* takes a rather different tack, following along on the assumption of the normality, as it were, of obsessive behavior. Macaulay makes the link that sees Johnson as a genius *because of* his afflictions and notes with a proto-Darwinian sense that Johnson "with such infirmities of body and mind" had to "fight his way through the world." Johnson's madness is now seen as a "hereditary malady," and Macaulay recognizes that "eccentricities less strange than his have often been thought grounds sufficient for absolving felons, and for setting aside wills."[96] Macaulay sees Johnson, from the perspective of the mid-nineteenth century, as having the kind of partial insanity that was by now accepted in courts of law. He notes that Johnson's symptoms "were the cruel marks left behind by a life which had been one long conflict with disease and adversity," but that, because Johnson was a genius with great faculties, he was always regarded with "interest" (31). When his friends thought him declining, his "strong faculties which had produced the *Dictionary* and *Rambler* were beginning to feel the effects of time and disease" (36). Macaulay says that they were wrong, and that his "failure was not to be ascribed to intellectual decay" (37).

Thus we can propose that the idea of partial madness as characteristic of humankind had become fairly well established by the beginning of the nineteenth century. Thomas Trotter, one of Cullen's students, taking off from his teacher's coinage of "neurosis," wrote about fifty years after Cheyne, "Sydenham at the conclusion of the seventeenth century, computed fevers to constitute two thirds of the diseases of mankind. But, at the beginning of the nineteenth century, we do not hesitate to affirm, that nervous disorders have now taken the place of fevers, and may be justly reckoned two thirds of the whole, with which civilized society is afflicted."[97]

When so many people, two-thirds of humanity, are seen as having nervous disorders, then we have entered the modern world characterized by what we might refer to as operative mental disorders, which allow people to both function and yet to think of themselves as mentally troubled.

EMERGENCE OF OBSESSION: THINKING
ABOUT ONE THING TOO MUCH

Here we see the emergence of the category of obsession. The condition does not yet have the name "obsession," but it emerges from between two models—it is both a type of mental illness and at the same time it is a cause of mental illness. Not a totalizing state, it is nonetheless a clearly defined state. We see the appearance of a condition of consciousness in which a person is obsessed by an idea, a series of thoughts, a person, or some other ruling passion but is otherwise lucid and is aware that some particular focus of attention is in play. Thus there is a conscious "I" who is watching an obsessed self instead of a deranged and unconscious self dwelling in a lunatic.

The nerve theory, unlike the quartet view of the body as a soupy cauldron of inner juices and vapors, allows for a single cause to create a slackening or a tightening of the nerves. A division between cause and effect, between parts affecting other parts, now replaces the previous totality of madness caused by the complex interactions of food, organs, humors, and juices. Now there is a sense that too much focus or a singleness of attention causes a problem. Nerves cause illness rather than the other way around. Cheyne started this concept rolling in the early part of the century when he wrote to Richardson and told him that his "sedentary life and thinking attentively" had caused his "wasted and relaxed nerves," and he recommended "keeping good hours, and never applying [that is, working] long at a time."[98] So Andrew Harper in 1789 could write that the cause of madness was a too fixed attention to specific things. He warns,

> But if the mental faculty happens to be particularly occupied and engaged by the presence and operation of some separate exclusive object, affection, or idea, or even peculiar train of uniform ideas, the mind, by being thus pitched upon a specific note and its nervous motions circumscribed within the limits of a certain modulation, receives too deep an impression, from this unchanging effect, in the tone of its movement.[99]

Here, nerves are conceptualized as being like catgut under tension in a stringed instrument. The mind can be put out of harmony by a tonic, in a musical sense, imbalance. As Harper continues,

Now this particular object, affection, or idea, thus in possession of the mental faculty, or prime movement, gains ground by continuance, and if it still remain in exercise, it gradually becomes the fixed, habitual motion, or predominant note, and then by engrossing the natural and general movements, it begins to obtund and interrupt the efficiency and perfection of the common and incidental ideas or impressions, and at last brings every image or modulation into unison with itself, and thus ultimately, by drawing the whole circle of sensorial motions into its own vortex, the order and harmony of mental operation is destroyed, and discord or insanity ensues. (34)

Harper pursues his notion that an obsession can create madness: "In every individual case of mania, without perhaps a single instance to the contrary, the torrent of the passions always flows in some particular channel, and the powers of the mind are chiefly spent upon one principal, overruling object" (34). Erasmus Darwin, forbear of both Charles Darwin and Francis Galton, wrote that "in every species of madness there is a peculiar idea either of desire or aversion, which is perpetually excited in the mind with all its connections. . . . So that the object of madness is generally a delirious idea, and thence cannot be conquered by reason."[100] Thomas Arnold, writing toward the end of the century, reminds us "that the ablest heads, and soundest judgments, may be deranged by too intense an application of mind."[101] He notes that thinking too much weakens the nervous system, interferes with digestion, and requires inactivity, late hours, and solitude.[102] Alexander Crichton, writing in 1798, tells us a similar thing, that an overexertion of mental faculties, particularly "a disproportionate activity of some of the said faculties; and the passions can cause mental derangement."[103]

Thus, the complexity of the humoral/organ theory gives way to the single-cause explanation—and in this case the single cause is too great a concentration on a single thing. Tissot, in his *An Essay on Diseases Incidental to Literary and Sedentary Persons,* translated into English in 1768, also rehearses the by now familiar dictum, which he traces from antiquity, that close study harms the body and the mind. Tissot, however, makes modern note of the role of brain and nerves in this process: "The head itself, and the nerves, and the stomach which is fuller of nerves than any other part, first suffer for the errors of the mind."[104] And he puts this point more directly when he writes, "Should it then seem surprising, if, when the tenor of the brain and nerves is broken by the efforts of the mind, the latter should decline in its turn?" (30). Reading, writing, and other intellectual activities, according to Tissot, when pursued diligently, can and do produce "nervous disorders" (34).

Nonmedical writers also accepted the idea that too strict attention to a specific thing could cause this new type of illness. Dr. Johnson in *Rasselas* has Imlac discuss this subject. Imlac takes note of the new expansion of madness to include obsessive and delusional states, nonclinical depression, and what later would be called, equally imprecisely, "neurosis."

> Disorders of intellect . . . happen much more often than superficial observers will easily believe. Perhaps, if we speak with rigorous exactness, no human mind is in its right state. There is no man whose imagination does not sometimes predominate over his reason, who can regulate his attention wholly by his will, and whose ideas will come and go at his command. No man will be found in whose mind airy notions do not sometimes tyrannize, and force him to hope or fear beyond the limits of sober probability.

Imlac goes on to say,

> All power of fancy over reason is a degree of insanity; but while this power is such as we can control and repress, it is not visible to others, nor considered as any depravation of the mental faculties: it is not pronounced madness but when it comes ungovernable, and apparently influences speech or action.[105]

Johnson's discussion points to the idea that all humans are to a degree mad in this new and partial way, an interesting fact given his own psychological state. What causes this "degree of insanity" is to be "too much in silent speculation." When that happens "in time some particular train of ideas fixes the attention, [and] all other intellectual gratifications are rejected." Then, "the mind, in weariness or leisure, recurs constantly to the favourite conception." Finally, "by degrees the reign of fancy is confirmed; she grows first imperious, and in time despotick. Then fictions begin to operate as realities, false opinions fasten upon the mind, and life passes in dreams of rapture or of anguish."[106]

Johnson's views are consistent with the ideas expressed at the time, that an excessive focus, what would be called an obsession or an idée fixe later on, causes this specifically new type of madness. Laurence Sterne, in the first two volumes of *Tristram Shandy* written in 1759, reminds us that concerning Uncle Toby's strange obsession with the battlefield of Namur, "when a man gives himself up to the government of a ruling passion,—or, in other words, when his Hobby-Horse grows headstrong,—farewell cool reason and fair discretion!"[107] Likewise, in Goethe's *The Sorrows of Young Werther* we see a portrait of the psyche of a man who eventually commits suicide over a fixed idea—his obsession with Lotte, who is inconveniently married to another man. Toward the climax of the novel, Lotte begs Werther to be more moderate and change his "fixed, uncontrollable passion."[108] The steady line of being too obsessed with an activity or a person leads to suicide and madness.

While not developing a full-blown theory of obsession, writers like Harper and Crichton are part of a continuum that begins to see "the fixed, habitual motion" or "predominant note" or "principal, over-ruling object" or "disproportionate activity" as a problem. An excessive focus on a particular activity or object can drive people mad, but mad in a way that is not totally mad. We recall that the mad people in *The Man of Feeling* all end up in Bedlam for obsessing too much on a subject rather than because of organic causes.

The idea of obsession treats the age-old concern over reason and passion in a new way. The Renaissance was concerned that reason dominate passions, as Castiglione advises in *The Book of the Courtier.* Likewise, classical eighteenth-century philosophy is signaled by its concern that reason predominate, as we see in Locke and Kant. But obsession is precisely the disease in which reason and passion exist on the same level. A passion exists and reason can speak about the passion, can observe the effect, but is powerless to stop the obsessive thought or action.

This attention to detail has another name, as we saw in *Caleb Williams*—curiosity. Curiosity, as Barbara Benedict tells us, is one of the hallmarks of eighteenth-century culture, which saw an uptick in collecting, cabinets of curiosities, connoisseurship, hobbyism, and so on.[109] The act of focusing intensely on one thing and collecting it had both a positive and a negative side, as Samuel Johnson noted in one of his *Rambler* essays. "Curiosity is the thirst of the soul; it inflames and torments us. . . . The desire of knowledge . . . seems on many occasions to operate without subordination to any other principle."[110] We seem to be looking at a transition from an interest in curiosity to a concern about obsession. Eighteenth-century habits of fascination and hobbyism, seen as eccentric, are now becoming a contributing cause of the newly invented category of mental illness. One early nineteenth-century writer complained that "one no longer says, it is his hobbyhorse (*dada*) his fancy (*marotte*). One says, like a grave physician, it is a monomania."[111]

Shortly after mid-eighteenth century, Tissot could write that "those are affected in the most dangerous manner, who dwell too long upon one and the same thought; for thus one part of the sensorium being longer stretch'd than the rest, without being ever reliev'd by the others in their turn, is the sooner broke."[112] And this line of reasoning continued through the early part of the nineteenth century as Sir Henry Holland wrote, "Certain cases of madness depend on a cause which can scarcely exist, even in slight degree without producing some mental disturbance: viz. *the too frequent and earnest direction of the mind inwards upon itself.*"[113] According to Michael J. Clarke, "morbid introspection" led to "the development of 'dominant,' 'imperative,' or obsessional ideas or trains of thought, of morbid emotional states, and of mental automatism, and thus by degrees passed over into actual mental disorder."[114]

This introspection is likely a product of a new culture of reading, philosophical speculation, and greater interest in the workings of the mind and the emotions. And here we have to ask ourselves whether we are seeing the beginning of a new disease entity alone or rather the beginning of an entirely new modality of thinking and being? What I will be suggesting throughout this work is that the distinction between disease and cultural activity is one that is hard to make, and that the making of that distinction is itself an act that is part of the process, not outside or tangential to that process.

What I have tried to show in this chapter is how the notion of obsession had to be established by the clearing of ground for the emergence of new cultural notions. The distinction between demonic possession and mental obsession had to be made. A notion of a partial insanity that was demotic in nature had to arise. The nerve theory had to be elaborated over the humoral/organ theory. The culture itself had to develop behaviors and ways of thinking that were repetitive, focused, and single-minded—and those behaviors had to be seen as both heuristic and at the same time dangerous. And the dangers had to become part of a cure system controlled by the emerging medical profession. All this had to happen, although not in any organized or even necessary way, so that obsession could come to the fore.

2

The Emergence of Obsession

MONOMANIA

By the early nineteenth century, beginning in France, the notion that the mind could be imbalanced or made unsound by a single idea or train of thought came to be called "monomania." This term, for all practical purposes, indicates the distinct emergence of the concept of, if not the term, obsession. The term "monomania" was introduced by Jean-Étienne Esquirol around 1810, preceded by Philippe Pinel's term "partial insanity," and was generally used to mean that only a single idea or faculty of the mind had been affected. By midcentury the idea was well accepted, as we can see by a summary article in a French medical journal that was translated and published in an American counterpart:

> We know that Pinel and Esquirol held it to be an incontestably established fact, has heretofore been but little disputed, that insanity may attack, partially, one or several of our faculties, without modifying, in any degree, the others, which remain intact as in a state of perfect health; in other words, that the insane person may reason justly upon all points, except that which is the constant object of his delirium.[1]

Monomania uses a structural view of the mind in which mental faculties, like branches of the university, are divided up, with most functioning while one or two are not fully operational. Monomania is defined as a disease in which monomaniacs are aware of the wrongness or inappropriateness of some aspect of their behavior, reasonably seeing that this function or action is awry, while still being able to use their reason to resist the action or thought. As the author of the summary article asks, "The question, as presented by M. Pinel, is, in fact, the one to be discussed: can insanity be partial, impairing some of our faculties to the exclusion of others so as to leave to us the appearances of reason whilst we really merit to be classed among the insane?"[2]

The significance of this diagnosis, as Simon During points out, is that "the peculiarity of monomania lay in its being (implicitly) a pathology of structure rather than content, so that the faculties themselves remained in order. Monomaniacs could 'think, reason, and act like other men.'"[3] If monomaniacs appear normal, and if there is difficulty in telling whether someone is a monomaniac or not, then the line between being normal and being insane becomes blurred indeed. This is of course the same definition as is used later in diseases like OCD, in which people can "think, reason, and act like other" people, but they are unable to stop a particular train of thought or action.

The diagnosis of monomania opened the doors to a wide-ranging application of the idea of insanity to the general population. Indeed, it is fair to say that at least in early nineteenth-century France the term "mania" was not the unique category it is today but rather was "the matrix species" through which Pinel and others viewed insanity, the "paradigmatic species of insanity that can shed light on all the others."[4] The number of people labeled lunatic in the nineteenth century went from a small fraction of the population at the beginning of the century to a rather large segment by the end. This was a phenomenon much commented upon by the medical profession and the public alike.[5] The number of nonhospitalized people who were considered mentally ill, particularly with the diagnosis of monomania, increased dramatically. After Esquirol invented the term, it became the single most frequently made diagnosis for patients entering the asylum at Charenton between 1826 and 1829 (when statistical records were kept), making up 45 percent of the inmate population. For the other famous asylums—Salpêtrière and Bicêtre—monomania diagnoses were the most common or second most commonly made.[6]

Like all the previous diagnoses we have seen, monomania would have a relatively short half-life, being dismissed toward the middle of the century and replaced by the newly redefined hysteria, neurosis, neurasthenia, and ultimately neurotic obsession and OCD. Yet monomania was the first diagnosis specifically defining what we are calling obsession. Further, perhaps because it defined something that had become culturally relevant and interesting, the general public, intellectuals, and novelists snatched it up in a relatively short time. Jan Goldstein points out that it took approximately a hundred and fifty years for the medical diagnosis of "nostalgia" to be adopted by the French Academy, while monomania required merely twenty-five years.[7] It was linked immediately with the notion of idée fixe, which was probably coined by phrenologists as they assimilated the concept of monomania. Monomania was defined as a preoccupation with a single idea, passion, or train of thought that was on the one hand obvious and knowable rationally to the subject while at the same time, despite the cognitive acknowledgment of the monomaniac, irresistible.

The diagnosis of monomania continues the trend of defining mental states not dependent on humors or thoracic organs to have produced them. It is a product of some vague combination of ideas and "nerves." To be sure, Esquirol saw monomania as a hybrid of melancholia (which he called lypemania) and mania. That is, melancholia, while totalizing, now is seen as allowing a self-awareness of one's depressed mood. Melancholia is no longer delusion. Pure mania was unaware, lost in its wild frenzy. But the new diagnosis of monomania, in effect, combined the awareness and the distraction in one entity.

Esquirol's definition of monomania was a "chronic cerebral affection, unattended by fever, and characterized by a partial lesion of the intelligence, affections or will."[8] This definition is worth noting because it places the provenance of monomania in the brain, along the nerve continuum, but refers to a "lesion" in a somewhat metaphysical way. Rather than an observable physiological lesion, this is what we might call a functional lesion. That is, there is a dysfunction of one of the faculties of the mind. These faculties, as described by Locke, are conceptual areas or functions of the brain like the ability to remember, to compare, or to abstract. This functional lesion leads to a situation in which "the intellectual disorder is confined to a single object," and "the patients seize upon a false principle, which they pursue without deviating from logical reasonings, and from which they deduce legitimate consequences, which modify their affections, and the acts of their will. Aside from this partial delirium, they think, reason and act, like other men."⁹ John Conolly's definition of insanity fits closely with Esquirol's definition of monomania: "Insanity . . . is the impairment of any one or more of the faculties of the mind, accompanied with, or inducing, a defect in the comparing faculty."¹⁰ In both definitions, only one thing is wrong—a "lesion" in either the faculty of reason or the faculty of comparison. Either way, it is a defect of rationality.

THE DISEASE OF CIVILIZATION; OR, WHEN A MAN'S SOUL GETS INTO HIS HEAD

In keeping with our notion that a general increase of the franchise on madness was taking place, monomania, at least in France, replaced the quartet, emphasizing the notion that this type of disease was in some sense deeply related to being civilized. Esquirol wrote that "monomania is, of all diseases, the one whose study offers the broadest and most profound subjects for meditation: the study of it embraces . . . that of civilization."¹¹ As Goldstein asserts, "According to Esquirol, the familiar propositions that 'madness is the disease of civilization' could be more correctly stated by substituting 'monomania' for 'madness.'"¹² Monomania, or what would later be called obsession, was thus seen as a quality of civilized life in which single ideas, thoughts, or emotions could derail, derange, the delicate balance of mind, body, and soul. This was a kind of insanity one could acquire in an almost random if not consumerist way. Indeed, Esquirol is quite specific about insanity in French women being caused by reading romances, attending the theater, listening to and playing music, and generally attending to society.¹³

Monomania was made a subject of popular discussion through some sensational trials in the nineteenth century in which seemingly ordinary people committed heinous crimes. Their defense was frequently made in the name of monomania. How else to explain the seeming randomness of a previously law-abiding and seemingly sane woman cutting off the head of a young child she barely knew, a man murdering and drinking the blood of his victim, and so on? These cases served well to expose the general public to the idea of monomania, which became itself a kind of obsession. One lawyer complained in 1828 that "we are 'monomanizing' (*monomaniser*) all the passions."¹⁴

As an example of how monomania caught on and became so integrated into the culture that it was a desirable thing, a state almost devoutly to be wished, we might observe the testimony of an anonymous American writer in 1856 who published an article entitled "Insanity—My Own Case" in the *American Journal of Insanity*. The writer is described by an editor as "a young gentleman of talent and literary pursuits"[15] who was a patient in the New York State Lunatic Asylum at Utica, New York. The author begins with a general disquisition on human nature in which he points out that "man, the most perfect and complicated in structure of all God's workmanship, is at the same time subject to the greatest number and variety of injurious agencies" (25). It is the complexity of humans, their god-likeness, that produces our ills, and so lunacy is seen as a result of the necessary and positive intricacy of being at the apex of creation. Insanity arises when this complex being comes into contact with "highly artificial modes of life" (25). The author makes a distinction between diseases of the body and of the mind. The latter affect the connection between the body and the mind and are called "nervous." He notes that the disease of the mind "has, till within a comparatively recent period, received little medical attention, probably because it has been thought incurable" (25–26). Observing pointedly that France leads the way in this area, he laments the difficulty of classifying mental diseases ("its types are so numerous and peculiar"), but he goes on to describe the accepted categories of mental illness—idiocy, total derangement of all the faculties, and finally "excessive activity or predominance of some particular faculty, sentiment, or propensity, or the entire occupation of the mind by some leading subject of thought till the perceptive powers become distorted with regard to all objects connected with that object, while they remain correct on all others" (26). This is clearly a description of monomania, and it is noteworthy that this intelligent patient has readily accepted the idea that "insanity often arises from excessive mental activity by which the nervous energy is withdrawn from the general system and concentrated in the brain" (27).

While the trigger for insanity is this devotion to excessive, single-minded, mental activity, that is, brain activity, the net result is a "disordered" nervous system. The nervous system is seen by this patient as "the connecting medium between mind and body" (26). This double nature of insanity, in which there is a somatic element and an ideational element, leads the author to see mental disease as "complex" and falling under both "physical or physiological" and "metaphysical" aspects and thus requiring treatment of both the material and spiritual aspects of the disease. In this case, the author was sent to the lunatic asylum following "protracted attendance" of his religious exercises.

The author rather beautifully refers to his obsession as a state of affairs "when a man's 'soul gets into his head'" (26). This is a disease of people with "large, active brains," and he notes sensibly that "a man should never become so scientific, so sentimental, or so religious, as to forget his dinner" (27). Physical symptoms like sleeplessness, loss of appetite, and lack of attention to the details of life come out of the idée fixe. "There is usually some leading idea, some ruling fantasy in the mind of an insane man, which is the cause of all his trouble" (28). Interestingly, the *OED* lists the first reference to "single-minded" in the sense of an adjective meaning focusing on a specific thing (rather than the older sense of steadfast) to 1860, the same time period in which this essay was written. The cure our patient notes for his disease is a purely mental one: "Let some one correct, rational idea be substituted in the place of a false one, and that, too, without sensibly disturbing the superstructure, like putting a new sill in a building, and it often paves the way for a gradual and complete recovery" (29). Recovery comes not from contradicting the person's obsession but by subtly and indirectly reshaping it. The author gives this example:

> For example, it is quite a common delusion with the insane that he is in the supernatural world; he loses all cognizance of time, and supposes eternity has commenced. In such a case there is but little use in denying this before him. He will believe you to be an emissary of Satan, sent to mislead and ruin his soul; but leave in his way a daily paper of a late date, or, if he be of a literary turn, a new book, by some favorite author, and the error will correct itself. (29)

DICKENS AS OBSERVER

Dickens's *American Notes,* written about a trip taken in 1842, recounts the author's visit to a hospital for the insane in South Boston which seems to follow the practices advocated above. Dickens is aware that the methods of this institution are new, following the ideas of moral treatment, rather than physical restraint and punishment, for insanity. The kind of madness depicted is almost exclusively of the monomaniacal variety. We meet Madge Wildfire, an inmate who believes she is a great, noble lady living in a royal mansion. The physician introduces Dickens to her, being sure to maintain the fiction of her nobility.

> "This," he said aloud, taking me by the hand and advancing to the fantastic figure with great politeness—not raising her suspicions by the slightest look or whisper, or any kind of aside to me: "This lady is the hostess of this mansion, sir. It belongs to her. Nobody else has anything whatever to do with it. It is a large establishment, as you see, and requires a great number of attendants. She lives, you observe, in the very first style."[16]

Dickens comments that the circle of madwomen "seemed to understand the joke perfectly (not only in this case, but in all the others, except their own) and to be highly amused by it." In this way he suggests that each woman, while able to see, and laugh at, the single error of Ms. Wildfire, and those of all the other madwomen in her company, is singularly unable to see her own delusion. And, as the anonymous author earlier suggested, Dickens notes that the physician at the hospital established so thorough a confidence that "opportunities are afforded for seizing any moment of reason to startle them by placing their own delusion before them." (240).

This rational and moral method is contrasted to an older-style "lunatic asylum" on Long Island, also visited by Dickens, that recalls the earlier corporeal methods of dealing with the insane. Gone is the respect and dignity, the "salutary system" of Boston, and what is left are physical restraints and mental disorder. Strangely present, to match the older system, are the older forms of madness. What Dickens sees is no longer this rather elegant and demotic form of monomania but the old intractable forms of idiocy and mania—"the moping idiot cowering down with long disheveled hair; the gibbering maniac with his hideous laugh and pointed finger; the vacant eye, the fierce wild face, the gloomy picking of the hands and lips; and munching the nails; there they were all, without disguise, in naked ugliness and horror" (290). Dickens leaves quickly saying, "The terrible crowd with which these halls and galleries were filled so shocked me that I abridged my stay within the shortest limits, and declined to see that portion of the building in which the refractory and violent were under closer restraint" (290). This scene is strangely reminiscent of the one in which Harley in Mackenzie's *Man of Feeling* visits Bedlam. Harley goes to see "the dismal mansions of those who are in the most horrid state of incurable madness," and laments that "the clanking of chains, the wild-ness of their [the inmates'] cries, and the imprecations which some of them uttered, formed a scene inexpressibly shocking."[17] Harley and his companions also begged their guide to leave the institution.

Dickens seems to be pointing back to the older forms of madness and the older forms of treatment. In Dickens's case we can see the more mod-ern sense of madness as monomania or obsession contrasted with the to-talizing form of madness. The modern form is not bathed in the pathos and disgust of the earlier manifestation. There is something alluring and indeed novelistic about these erring players who see themselves in a role that they don't quite understand. There is a wink and a nod, a communal sense of the irrational, that contrast sharply with the filth and despair of the antiquated form of madness.

MONOMANIA IN *FRANKENSTEIN*

It is no surprise that the concept of monomania, therefore, took to lit-erature and culture like wildfire. Perhaps the first and most obvious use was in the classic work of obsession—Mary Shelley's *Frankenstein,* which she began writing in 1816. Not uncoincidentally, Shelley's father was Wil-liam Godwin, author of *Caleb Williams,* and her mother was Mary Woll-stonecraft, author of *Maria*—both works with strong elements of the obsessive. In *Frankenstein,* the central characters are all men with obses-sions of the monomaniacal type. Captain Walton is obsessed with finding the North Pole, Victor Frankenstein with creating life, and the monster with revenge. All of them share the fact that their lives are devoted to an idée fixe. And each becomes deranged by his exclusive focus on his goal. Walton begins his account with a description of his "ardent curiosity" to make a scientific discovery by going to find the North Pole. In some ways, Walton is the poster boy for monomania. He is "passionately fond of reading," has a "passionate enthusiasm" for the ocean, and believes, incorrectly, that "nothing contributes so much to tranquillise the mind as a steady purpose—a point on which the soul may fix its intellectual eye."[18] His focus is intense and desperate, we note, as he says, "Gladly I would sacrifice my fortune, my existence, my every hope, to the furtherance of my enterprise" (28).

When Walton picks up the shipwrecked Victor Frankenstein, the for-mer immediately sees in the latter a peer of this obsessive realm, someone with whom he can "sympathise" (19, 21). At this point, the end of the story although the beginning of the novel, Victor Frankenstein's sole idea is "to seek one who fled from me" (26), an interesting echo of Caleb Williams's own idée fixe. The connection between Frankenstein and Walton is immediate and understandable to both. Frankenstein says with high emotion, in tears and quivering, "Unhappy man. Do you share my madness? Have you drank also of the intoxicating draught? Hear me,—let me reveal my tale, and you will dash the cup from your lip" (28). Frankenstein, by now, is already "mad," but he wishes to discourage Walton from the same obsessive pursuit of a single idea. As he cautions, "Learn from me, if not by my precepts, at least by my example, how dangerous is the acquirement of knowledge" (53). Frankenstein, when he recounts his own biography, "the vision of a madman" (52), dwells on his single-minded pursuit of knowledge. He had a desire to learn, but not to learn "all things indiscriminately." Rather than being a Renaissance man or a proponent of the liberal arts, Victor explains that he had focused exclusively on "the physical secrets of the world." In doing so, he was attacked by a "passion, which afterwards ruled my destiny," obliterating his carefree childhood, replacing it with a "misfortune" that tainted his mind and "changed its bright visions of extensive usefulness into gloomy and narrow reflections upon self" (37–38). There was a woeful fall from a romantic world of childhood filled with possibility to the narrow and dark world of obsession, so that "my mind was filled with one thought, one conception, one purpose" (48).

That madness has a name, and it is "science." Frankenstein says that in the liberal arts "you go as far as others have gone before you, and there is nothing more to know; but in a scientific pursuit there is continual food for discovery and wonder." While there are benefits to this kind of study, Frankenstein will become an example of how he "sought the attainment of one object of pursuit, and was solely wrapt up in this." (51). We see the repetition of the motif "one pursuit" throughout Frankenstein's narrative[19] with the accompanying sense of irresistible attraction, as in, "I could not tear my thoughts from my employment" (55).

What Shelley is presenting, in the form of Frankenstein's obsession, is the nerve-induced monomania that we have seen in the writings of mad doctors. The presentation is more like something that belongs in medical texts than in a novel. Frankenstein discusses the metaphysical issue saying, "A human being in perfection ought always to preserve a calm and peaceful mind, and never to allow passion or a transitory desire to disturb his tranquility. I do not think the pursuit of knowledge is an exception to this rule." Shelley, through Victor, characterizes this kind of study, which weakens human affections and destroys the simple pleasures of life, as "unlawful" and "not befitting the human mind" (56). The result was that Victor "became nervous to a most painful degree," which he himself sees as the signs of "incipient disease" (56). The symptoms of this disease are even described—rapid pulse, languor, and extreme weakness, excess sensitivity to touch and to stimuli, wildness, and loud, unrestrained laughter caused by being "so deeply engaged in one occupation" (58–59, 61). All of these are precursors to "a nervous fever" (62) that overtakes Frankenstein after he has created his monster.

The end of the story appears to be an even stronger statement on the hazards of an idée fixe. The crew of Walton's ship stages a mutiny and refuses to go on. Frankenstein advises Walton to continue, and even addresses the mutinous men using the language of single-mindedness: "Are you then so easily turned from your design. . . . Be steady to your purposes" (214–15). When Walton decides to honor his crew's request and turn back, Frankenstein says ruefully, "Do so, if you will; but I will not. You may give up your purpose, but mine is assigned to me by Heaven" (216). So it is only Walton who abandons his cause and, as a result, remains the only sane one of the three. By the end of the story, the monster appears to commit suicide, Frankenstein dies on Walton's ship, and Walton endures.

BALZAC AND IDÉE FIXE

One can see much of nineteenth-century fiction as theme and variation on monomania. Balzac's *Old Goriot,* published in 1834, about fifteen years after *Frankenstein,* is the story of an obsessive monomaniac—Old Goriot is so devoted to this two spoiled daughters that he gives up everything, including his life, for the satisfaction of their needs. Balzac was well aware of Esquirol's writings on monomania, and thought to use the concept as an informing armature for this early novel. Indeed, Balzac himself was an obsessive hoarder and collector, as was one of his later characters Cousin Pons.[20] As Vautrin, the criminal, says in explaining Goriot's behavior, "Well . . . these people get their teeth into one idea and you can't shake them loose from it. They are thirsty, but only for water taken from one particular well. . . . For some men this well is gambling, speculation on the stock exchange, or it may be music or a collection of pictures or insects.

For others it is a woman."[21] We familiarly note the classic description of an idée fixe. At Goriot's demise, Bianchon, a young medical student, observes the old man, of whom he says, "He thinks of nothing but his daughters." Bianchon is told by his supervising doctor to note that the patient "should show particular preoccupations according to the region of the brain affected by the pressure of serum." And the medical student advises Bianchon to "note to what category of ideas what he says belongs; whether he uses his memory, or his powers of perception or judgement; whether his thoughts are concerned with material matters or feelings; whether he plans for the future, or returns to the past; in short, be prepared to give us an exact report." In other words, Bianchon is to conduct an experiment on Goriot to ascertain which faculty of his mind has a lesion.

SPECIALIZATION AS OBSESSION

While Goriot is not a particularly intellectual man, he illustrates some of the stresses of living life in the fast track in a complex and pressured society. But Esquirol and others came to link monomania and other forms of insanity with the very things that we would now praise as the best things produced by civilization—art and learning. The rise of specialization and professionalism are characteristic of the eighteenth and nineteenth centuries. The older idea of the Renaissance man or woman whose fame comes from the variety of his or her knowledge gives way to the expert with a single focus. Of course, the polymath and the multitalented genius might indeed have lived on in various forms, but the new zeitgeist emphasized the person who was the "novelist" or the "composer" or the "medical man" or even the "mad doctor," the "alienist," and so on. Along with this change to specialization came the growth of professional organizations and the establishment of the modern university with its own "faculties" that shared, in effect, notions of the faculties of the mind. The model provided by Locke of a mind with various faculties—perception, comparison, memory, and so on—became a model for the more general structure and function of thinking or understanding.

Society at large became, to an extent, monomaniacal in the way that it emphasized specialization and the development of particular faculties. The question then became a larger one in the nineteenth century—can humans specialize and develop specific knowledges without becoming obsessed or insane? Did faculties, on both the large and small scales, become "unbalanced" when one of the faculties was overly stressed or relied upon? Did the advancement of civilization lead inevitably to nervousness and madness?

Esquirol had to take on this question. His answer was that some "men of genius," of great intellectual capacity, were not predisposed to insanity. Yet those people were few, while "the greater part of painters, also of poets and musicians, impelled by the need of emotions, abandon themselves to numerous errors of regimen."[22] And in the case of scholars of lesser capacity, "the understanding takes an exclusive direction; and the man meditates without cessation, upon subjects connected with metaphysical speculations, and confines himself to them, with a determination proportionate to the efforts that are made to divert his mind. . . . He neglects the most important personal attentions, condemning himself to practices which seriously affect his constitution."[23] This kind of monomania is not simply confined to individuals but can replicate itself on cultures at large so that entire cultures can become monomaniacal. Philippe Pinel wrote that "so many causes, in the large cities, are present to produce and foment the nervous illnesses! The spread of enervating luxury, of an inactive and sedentary life style . . . continued use of carriages, the use of fermented liquors . . . the torments of ambition, dissipation, pleasure."[24]

Obsession and monomania come together in the sense that an idée fixe becomes an inescapable reality. As Esquirol notes, "All monomaniacs . . . are pursued both night and day, by the same thoughts and affections, which are the more disordered as they are concentrated or exasperated by opposition."[25] Thus obsession becomes a distinct category of existence, and one often linked to being an artist, a writer, a scientist—in short, a specialist.

We must also think of the link, not the separation, between the mad doctor and the mad patient. As contemporaries understood, the development of science, and medical science in particular, was not unrelated to the new kind of madness we have been discussing. Samuel Tissot writing in 1767 creates a sort of memorial within his work to a friend who bore in his being the contradiction between these definitions of science and obsession:

I must still grieve for a friend of penetrating genius, an excellent understanding, of strict morals, and one that seem'd born for a better fate; who being animated with too great a love of learning, and in particular of the medical science, by reading night and day, observing, making experiments, and meditating, at first became sleepless; then began to talk, sometimes incoherently, and sometimes rationally; at last run mad, and having scarcely escap'd with life, never recovr'd his reason.[26]

Tissot sees this type of overwork as endemic to the project of science and study. He allows for a few great people like Descartes, Newton, or Montesquieu who have had the fortitude to engage in sustained study. But reacting to the vogue for specialization and learning that goes under the name of science, he cautions, "Most studious men lose their time, and break their constitutions to no purpose; one makes a collection of common-place topicks, another embellishes such as are threadbare, a third anxiously investigates matters of no utility, others make trifles the subject of laborious researches, and all are equally unmindful of the unprofitableness and danger of their pursuits."[27] While there is tradition carrying back to Burton that notes the diseases of the learned, there is a distinct change here that specifically makes a connection between the diseases of attention and the professions that exist because of attention.

In this chapter we have seen how monomania paved the way for obsessive diseases, obsessive practices, and a general culture of attention, focus, specialization—all of these linked to the rise of professions and science. There was no necessity that these features would coalesce into a culture of obsession, but there seems to be a trend, a river made up converging streams, a zeitgeist within a culture, that leads to both the concept of scientific observation and its dark side, the diseases of hyperattention and obsessive focus.

3

Specialization as Monomania

We might be able to use this notion of an expanded class of people with madness as a kind of portal into modernity. It has been notoriously difficult to assign a definition to modernity, and so I don't think I will make much headway in that endeavor. Yet I would like to put forward the idea that modernity may be seen as a period in which the normal state of being is defined as allied with being somewhat mad, and particularly with being obsessed.[1] The form of this obsession is a singular attention to a particular thing or things, which in effect is the definition of specialization—itself an acknowledged feature of modernity.

In a philosophical sense, this new notion of the alienated mind as characteristic of human subjectivity places us in a special situation *vis à vis* subjectivity and identity. The mind that increasingly is postulated by the Enlightenment is one that can observe itself. It is in this sense alienated from itself. Indeed, it is the very Lockean idea of the mind observing its succession of images and thoughts that gives rise to a definition of being as awareness. The mind of the insane had therefore been formerly postulated as closed to subjectivity and intersubjectivity—that is unavailable to reason and self-reason. But Locke views the mind not as a monolithic soul given by God and therefore totalized with either sanity or madness,

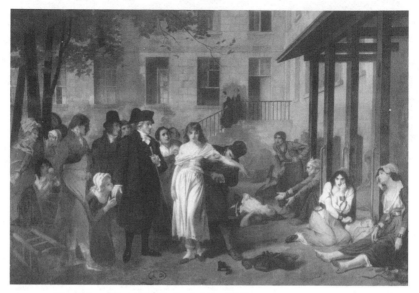

FIGURE 4. Tony Robert-Fleury, *Pinel Freeing the Insane* (1876).

virtue or sin, but as a loose amalgamation of states of mind which interact with each other. This view allows for a new view of consciousness and affect. With the advent of the idea of obsession as a semi-rational state, the mind is redefined along these Lockean and Kantian terms as composed of rational faculties, most particularly the faculty of comparison. These newly defined insane people are able rationally to compare their faculties, although there may be an error in one or more of these faculties. According to Marcel Gauchet and Gladys Swain, this opening up allows for the idea of curability, which Pinel introduces or elaborates in France at the beginning of the nineteenth century. Curability speaks of a subjectivity which is not eradicated, as earlier views of madness might have had it.[2] Curability, in turn, becomes a sign of Enlightenment. Nothing is more touching than the idea of Pinel liberating the inmates of the insane asylum from their chains, even if, according to some, they went from chains to straitjackets (fig. 4).

Chains, as it were, do not bind the Enlightenment mind, as William Blake illustrated in his paintings, but that mind was free to recover with the help of a progressive state. In France, the revolution led almost immediately to the reformulation of ideas about madness and cure. This changeover should alert us immediately to the inherently political nature of metaphors of the mind and madness. In a democratic environment, there would be no use for a subjectivity that was isolated and unavailable to itself. So, rather, the project had to be twofold: the expansion of the category of madness—particular the kind in which one faculty was out of line with all the others—so that this obsessiveness became a characteristic of humanity; and second, the inevitable notion that insanity was curable through humane means involving moral treatment and direct discourse rather than isolation and physical restraint. Curability, also, has a strong implication that science, in this case medicine, has a great power. It is not ineffective against madness. Curability then becomes the medical version of that famous nineteenth-century word—progress.

It is noteworthy too that ideas of normality had to come into play. As I have demonstrated in *Enforcing Normalcy* and *Bending Over Backwards,* the very concept of the norm was tied up with the development of paradoxically a eugenics movement and also a progressive and democratic agenda. The issues around cognitive and affective disorders also follow this schema. The eugenic impulse to improve and better humankind is immediately found in Pinel and Esquirol's work in France as well as in the moral treatment movement in England and elsewhere. Yet this same impulse also creates a new category of human—the disabled, the deformed, the hereditary insane. The asylum movement aims to relieve the ordinary human of his or her problems at the same time that it ends up incarcerating and isolating such people. The nineteenth century reveals a medicalized history that places the insane person squarely within the domestic sphere as the hysterical housewife, the masturbating adolescent, the nervous patient, the neurasthenic citizen, while at the same time indicating that the condition was paradoxically both curable and yet chronically resistant to cure. Simultaneously, the mind is seen as radically material—composed of brain, nerves, and lesions—while also being overtly immaterial and thought-driven. And then there is some combination of both—the mind that is capable of being mesmerized, magnetized, hypnotized into denying exterior reality or even communicating with spirits.

It will be necessary to think about obsession as a kind of hyperattention to specialization. It would then apply not only to the patient but to the physician observer of that class of patients. Obsession sits on both sides of the consulting table. In addition, we might consider the modernity of the city with its increasingly regularized space, regulated timetables for public transportation, standardization of building practices, and so on as another instance of obsessive attention to detail. In addition, one might consider the rise of the modern university, with its categorization of knowledge, as well as the rise of science, with its concomitant practices of statistics. Indeed, it could be argued that these practices constitute the social and cultural formations of modernity. Likewise, the stress deriving from living this kind of increasingly specialized and regulated existence creates and necessitates a life of obsessive activity. This latter kind of obsession is seen both as fitting into modernity and paying the price for modernity. The nervous exhaustion that is the metaphor behind neurasthenia, the repetitive activity of the mind in mental breakdown, the fixed notions that characterize the "shattered" nerves and enervated brain of the nineteenth century are the products and results of modernity as a lived experience.

PEACOCK ON BLACK BILE AND SCIENCE

Thomas Love Peacock's rather strange book *Nightmare Abbey*, published in 1818, provides us with a window into this phenomenon. His work is a satire on the times, in which he sees the characteristic mental and emotional life as one vastly altered from that of his forbears. In a letter to Percy Bysshe Shelley, he notes that he wrote the novel to "'make a stand' against the 'encroachments' of black bile . . . to bring a sort of philosophical focus of a few of the morbidities of modern literature and to let a little daylight on its atrabilarious complexion." Peacock is complaining about the tendency he sees in his contemporaries to adopt the mental maladies, most particularly depression, as a way of life. Modern existence is, from his point of view, integrated with issues of mental disorder. He opens the novel with a quote from Samuel Butler which begins, "There's a dark lantern of the spirit," as well as one from Ben Jonson about the relation between melancholy and wit. The opening lines introduce the father of the main character, Scythrop, who is characterized as being of an "atrabilarious" temperament and "much troubled with those phantoms of indigestion which are commonly called 'blue devils.'"[3] Scythrop (whose name means "gloomy face") is supposed to be Shelley himself. He goes about with a copy of Goethe's *Sorrows of Young Werther,* a book itself about melancholy and monomania, most particularly erotomania. Scythrop also has William Godwin's *Mandeville* in his library, which one character describes as "the morbid anatomy of black bile" (60). Characters in the novel continually lament "My nerves . . . my nerves are shattered" (59). The nervous system is invoked when another character notes that "tea has shattered our nerves; late dinners make us slaves of indigestion" (68). And more conclusively another character laments that there is "a conspiracy against cheerfulness. . . . How can we be cheerful when our nerves are shattered" (103).

Peacock's novel is a dialogue between characters who are satiric stand-ins for Byron, Shelley, Mary Shelley, Coleridge, and other recognizable cultural figures of the day, which makes the general assessments of the time somewhat more compelling. One of the most significant rants comes from Mr. Asterias, who represents science and complains of the prevalence of the quartet: "spleen, chagrin, vapours, blue devils . . . have infected society." He does not see (and how could he?) that science is part of this series of infections, although Peacock's aim is to satirize his alternative to the quartet. Asterias's obsession is tied to his specialization of ichthyology, and his supposedly disinterested approach to nature leads to his gullibly rushing to the seaside on the report of a mermaid sighting. He complains that "splenetic and railing misanthropy" is the current mode in which "speculative energy" takes form, and contrasts his own "calm dignity" and "disinterested pleasures of enlarging intellect" as the scientist. Yet the satire points us toward the conclusion that, as one character says, "the devil has come among us and has begun by taking possession of all the cleverest fellows" (100).

Science, with its obsessive focus, is the means by which individuals reshape the biosphere and at the same time pay the price for that obsession. Although we are used to an idea of science as integrated easily into our lives, we have to imagine how strange the notion of science was to someone at the beginning of the nineteenth century, and how much stranger were the people who were collecting specimens and performing experiments. A poem to science written by Sarah Hoare, published in 1831, apostrophizes science as an "illuminating ray, fair mental beam."[4] The intensity of that idea of focus, on a searing visual focus, characterizes the way people might have thought about science. Indeed, one of the hallmarks of this practice, particularly on the part of those studying madness, was an attention to measurement, cataloging, taxonomies, and informal types of experimentation.[5] As G. Berrios notes,

Early nineteenth-century alienists inherited a set of molar categories (mania, melancholia, phrensy, lethargy, etc.) the semantic bounds of which were strongly determined by social variables. By the end of the century some of these categories had gone for good, others had been drastically refurbished and yet others created anew. More importantly, the semantic bounds of the new categories were now determined by empirical rules obtained directly from observation and counting.[6]

Observation and counting might be said to be two behaviors that characterize the new "rigors" of science and medicine. Charts, graphs, tables seem to convey a kind of mathematical reassurance that the phenomena studied are actually what Dickens had called, ironically, "hard facts." But counting and observation of a particular kind are what we also associate with obsessive behaviors. Indeed, scientists were from the beginning seen as oddballs. As Thomas Peacock's novel indicates, his scientist is a strange person with a stranger obsession. Later in the century, a family member characterized Luke Howard, the meteorological cataloger of cloud types, as "a sensitive man, with a good deal of the oddity of genius, and its waywardness."[7] The nature of the oddity was that he "seemed always to be thinking of something very far away. . . . He was often contemplating the weather and would stand for a long time at the window gazing at the sky with his dreamy placid look, occasionally drawing our attention to some grand cloud, and explaining its form."[8]

SIR FRANCIS GALTON: OBSESSIVE CASE IN POINT

It might be instructive to look extensively at a particular individual who, we might say, is typical of his time, who illustrates through lived experience the kinds of complex relations to self, career, and psyche that were becoming a new kind of norm for existence, a norm of the obsessional, particularly in science. Sir Francis Galton was born in 1822 in Birmingham. He is best known as the founder of eugenics and was also an early statistician. Through his own recollections in his memoirs, we get an insight into Galton. The first thing to note is that Galton—unlike a fellow memoirist like Rousseau—has taken a "scientific" view of his own life. Characteristically, Galton chose to organize his book in a kind of statistical way, as he writes:

These "Memories" are arranged under the subjects to which they refer, and only partially in chronological order. A copious list of my memoirs will be found in the Appendix with dates attached to them. These show what inquiries were going on at or about any specified year. The titles of books are printed in heavy letters. They summarize, as a rule, the best parts of the corresponding memoirs up to the dates of their publication.[9]

It is telling that, for Galton, the mechanics of the arrangement of the book come before anything else. Rather than choosing the logic of chronology, the time-honored way to recount the story of one's life, Galton will arrange events by "subject," but allow for an appendix that will retain the chronological approach along with the nosological. In addition, he adds that "the method of that most useful volume," the *Index and Epitome of the Dictionary of National Biography,* will be used in listing the birth and death dates of each person mentioned. So, for Galton, a life is more like a dictionary, in effect, than a novel.

According to Galton's own testimony, his attention to this kind of detail, this obsession with order and cataloging, was hereditary. His grandfather "was a scientific and statistical man of business" with "a decidedly statistical bent, loving to arrange all kinds of data in parallel lines of corresponding lengths, and frequently using colour for distinction."[10] His father was also "eminently statistical by disposition."[11] As the founder of eugenics, Galton naturally embraced the notion of inherited traits, and he mentions that his father and his siblings "inherited this taste in greater or lesser degree." Of greater degree was his aunt, who acquired numbers of blank books, neatly ruled them with red ink, assigned them some year and function, and filled them with notations in color "with little reason, but with regard to their pictorial effect" (3). Galton continued along with her obsession by collecting his aunt's books after her death "as a psychological curiosity."

The notion of an order that must be kept is linked to Galton's own notions of heredity, the process that preserves order over generations. Although Galton's ideas of heredity do not correspond to what we now know about the actual way that traits are passed along, they nevertheless express the will and desire that an orderly line of inheritance inform human life. Thus Galton could write that he "acknowledge[s] the debt to my progenitors of a considerable taste for science, for poetry, and for statistics." He also traces various diseases back to his relatives (11). It is possible for us to conjecture that the fascination of the nineteenth century with hereditarian explanations comes from a distinctly obsessive notion that history, even biological history, is orderly, keeping and maintaining the traits of past progenitors. In fact, genetic inheritance is a good deal messier, without the one-for-one correspondence that the nineteenth century assumed about traits and bloodlines.

In keeping with the cultural models of madness I've been tracing, and perhaps as a consequence of his obsessions and focused attentions, Galton developed various mental maladies. His attitude toward his "illness" is consistent with the new view we have seen that madness is connected with being human, and that genius and madness are close cousins. Of this fact, Galton laments, "Poor humanity! I often feel that the tableland of sanity upon which most of us dwell, is small in area, with unfenced precipices on every side, over any one of which we may fall" (38). Indeed, in his third year at Oxford, Galton "broke down entirely in health" and had to return home for a term. Galton describes his symptoms: "I suffered from intermittent pulse and a variety of brain symptoms of an alarming kind. A mill seemed to be working inside my head; I could not banish obsessing ideas; at times I could hardly read a book, and found it painful even to look at a printed page" (78). It's noteworthy that this is the first explicit use of "obsessing ideas" that we have seen in this study. Galton's explanation for this disease that could have become "madness" was "I had been much too zealous, had worked too irregularly in too many directions, and had done myself harm" (78). Galton makes the analogy between his own physical system and that of a steam engine both in his reference to the "mill" working in his head and in the following: "It was as though I had tried to make a steam-engine perform more work than it was constructed for, by tampering with its safety valve and thereby straining its mechanism" (79). The by-now standard midcentury explanation of neurasthenia is presented here with the familiar analogy of a modern machine being overworked or depleted of energy. Indeed, the word "break-down," according to the *OED* was first used for machinery in 1838, followed in twenty years for mental or physical health.[12]

Galton recovered, but, later in life when he married, he again had "a more serious breakdown than had happened before." He "suffered" during the thirteen years following his marriage in 1853 from "giddiness and other maladies prejudicial to mental effort." Following the standard prescription for neurasthenia of ceasing mental activities and increasing exercise and fresh air, he "invariably became well again." But in 1866 he had a more serious breakdown. Notably, Galton says that his symptoms were "small problems, which successively obsessed me day and night, as I tried in vain to think them out. These affected mere twigs, so to speak, rather than large boughs of the mental process, but for all that most painfully."[13] Again, using directly the language of obsession, Galton is saying that he wasn't crazy writ large, but crazy in lowercase — the major functions of his brain were not affected, only the smaller functions. But the diminishment of these functions, the obsessive, repetitive ones that affected process rather than content, was nonetheless painful and problematic. In other words, Galton is acknowledging the kind of obsessive disorder that we have seen as characterized by being partial — the consumerist, democratic kind of breakdown that links the possessor with all the other hardworking, intelligent, neurasthenics who make up the ruling and cultural elites of the country.

Galton's tendency toward obsessive thinking caused his breakdowns, according to his view, but we should also note that the same tendency, in effect, made him a scientist in his own era. There are several ways we could think about this issue. One would be to say that a mode of thinking, or a way of thinking about thinking, arises in a certain era in particular cultures and that this mode is then simultaneously elevated to a cultural goal and also problematized as a medical or even criminal problem. In this case, we have seen that obsessional thinking, the focusing on one subject, the schematic measuring and charting of life activities or physical dimensions, the repetitive and ruminative thinking on a particular subject, led in at least two directions — the first toward the scientific method and the second toward the disease entities of obsession, monomania, idée fixe. As would also be the case, these latter became the object of study of the former. Galton's own life embodies this split, which also includes the rise of the modern forms of discursive oppressions — eugenics, the rise of racial science, discourses of surveillance, colonialism, and so on — in all of which Galton was intimately involved. Galton founded eugenics, helped to provide statistics on racial stereotypes, invented fingerprinting, "discovered," mapped, and claimed areas of South Africa, and even ended up being the director of the Kew Observatory, where he helped to standardize the calibration of scientific tools for time measurement. At the same time, Galton's activities led him to take on the symptoms available for nineteenth-century mental disabilities—neurasthenia, mental break-down, and hysteria—manifested in the form of obsessional thinking and compulsive activity.

To see this point more clearly, let us look at some of Galton's scientific endeavors. In many of these, we can see personal interest, daily life, and observation shading into obsessive thinking and compulsive activity that also might be called scientific research. Take an article that Galton published in *Nature* that began with an observation.

> A curious sight caught my attention on one of these occasions [at the race track]. I was on the side of the course that faced the distant [viewing] stand, and amused myself while waiting in studying the prevalent tint of the faces upon it. At length the horses were off, but it was hot, and I was contented to remain in quiet where I was. When the horses approached the winning post, the prevalent tint of the faces in the great stand changed notably, and became distinctly more pink under the flush of entertainment. (179)

Galton's proclivity toward the statistical allows him to observe details of lived experience that had not been, historically, subject to this type of analysis. Indeed, it is reasonable to suppose that a human being measuring the tint of the faces in a crowd might have been thought very eccentric in an earlier, nonscientific, time. Also the results of such observation would probably not have been put into print.

In effect, what we are witnessing in this period is the tendency to include the human in the study of nature. Certainly, in the eighteenth century and earlier, science involved the "discovery" and charting of natural phenomena, including mapping the world, measuring distances, stan-dardizing time, setting up taxonomies of genus and species of fauna and flora, as well as chemicals, geology, and so on. But the nineteenth century saw the inclusion of the human into the measurement of nature. There are complex explanations for this change, including the dethroning of humans from a kind of divinely ordained sovereignty over nature. While Renaissance philosophers like Pico della Mirandola had seen humans as the pinnacle of the divine creation, and eighteenth-century philosophers like Vico had acknowledged the secular nature of human history, the nineteenth century finally arrived at a placement of humans well within the natural world, so that humans were capable of being studied as one might study the life and times of the mollusk. This revelation became a true obsession, so that the statistical measurement of human physiology and capacity, as well as the determination to find clear mental and affective paradigms, dominated the intellectual life of the nineteenth century. People like Galton, whose measuring obsession might well have been deemed insane in a previous century, certainly worthy of inhabiting Swift's Academy of Lagado in *Gulliver's Travels,* are now looked upon as engaged in a worthwhile activity.

Another example of Galton's research might be useful here. Galton, having decided that "many mental processes admit of being roughly measured," decided to measure human boredom by counting the number of times a group of people fidgeted. As a member of the Royal Geographical Society, he had the occasion to observe attendees at the meetings of that august organization, where, as Galton wryly notes, "even there dull memoirs are occasionally read." His scientific method was to choose a section of two or three rows in the observer gallery bounded by two wrought iron pillars as a "convenient sample." Galton would count the number of fidgets per group per minute and then calculate the average number of fidgets per person. To create a truly scientific experiment in which the observer would not be observed, he invented a technique for measuring time, since "the use of a watch attracts attention, so I reckon time by the number of my breathings, of which there are fifteen in a minute. They are not counted mentally, but are punctuated by pressing with fifteen fingers successively. The counting is reserved for the fidgets" (278). What seems like a very difficult and annoying process of "scientific" observation is for Galton an activity that "I have often amused myself with." Here we have Galton both counting his own breaths on his fingers, and mentally or on paper the number of fidgets per minute, to attain a "scientific" result. This obsessive-compulsive activity now serves the interest of scientific progress and comes to be printed in a scientific journal without comment on its perhaps obsessive nature. Science is what one deliberately does; obsession is what one can't help doing—a nice distinction that collapses frequently.

It is no coincidence that Galton's attention to his own breathing became, in turn, a subject for a further obsession. Here the scientific crosses over into the personal and indeed obsessional. Galton recalls that "in the days of my youth I felt at one time a passionate desire to subjugate the body by the spirit, and among other disciplines determined that my will should replace automatism by hastening or retarding automatic acts." To do so, he became hyperaware of his own breathing, and he attempted to make every breath a conscious act. As a result, not surprisingly, "every breath was submitted to this process, with the result that the normal power of breathing was dangerously interfered with" (276).

Another invention still furthered his obsessive attention to breathing. He experimented with the sensation of suffocation and was "surprised at the absence of that gaping desire for air" that most people report feeling. Galton notes that he felt ill at the point of fainting, but nothing more.[14] Galton then had prescription goggle-glasses made for him so he could "read the print of a newspaper perfectly under water." Engaged in such activity, "I amused myself very frequently with this new hobby, and being most interested in the act of reading, constantly forgot that I was nearly suffocating myself."[15] Retrospectively, we can surmise that Galton's scientific interest was in effect a kind of hyperawareness of bodily states that might be characterized as a form of obsessive-compulsive disorder.

Galton's minute measurements of his own body and the bodies of others were in keeping with his own general eugenic and statistical projects. He describes "the pressing necessity of obtaining a multitude of exact measurements relating to every measurable faculty of body or mind, for two generations at least, on which to theorise" (244). This project would have been almost unimaginable a century earlier. The activity of mapping, detailing, cataloging, organizing the biosphere is characteristic of Galton and his era, as well as ours. Galton even went so far as to assemble data for a "Beauty-Map" of the British Isles. Again, the obsessive-compulsive prevails. Galton notes that whenever he meets people, "I have occasion to classify the persons I meet into three classes, 'good, medium, bad.'" On his walks through a city, he would take a piece of paper, write the place and date on it, and tear it into a cross, using a needle to prick holes in the paper cross "upper end for 'good,' the cross-arm for 'medium,' the lower end for 'bad.'" Then Galton would walk along "classifying the girls I passed on the streets or elsewhere as attractive, indifferent, or repellent." His categories may have been a bit simplistic, and he admits that "this was a purely individual estimate," but he notes that although personal, "it was consistent, judging from the conformity of different attempts in the same population." The results were that London ranked the highest for beauty and Aberdeen the lowest (315).

The low ranking for Scotland may have been related to Galton's ideas about race and racial superiority, with London being the center and apex of all things hereditary while Scotland was seen as less developed. The way that Galton applied his obsessive attention to women through the modality of the statistical is demonstrated by another remarkable racialized moment. Galton traveled extensively through South Africa and had received a gold medal from the Royal Geographical Society "for having . . . fitted out an expedition . . . to a country hitherto unknown . . . a country never before penetrated by a civilized being" (150). In the process of penetrating this country, Galton, according to his biographer, ran into a "Hottentot Venus." The biographer's reference harks back to Saartjie Baartman, an African woman known as the "Hottentot Venus" who was exhibited as a "freak" in London in 1810, and was known mainly for the large proportions of her steatopygian buttocks. Galton's initial response as a "scientific man" to this beautiful African woman was that he was "exceedingly anxious to obtain accurate measurements of her shape," by which we presume he wanted to measure the size of her buttocks. Galton notes that since he didn't speak the language, he could "never therefore have explained to the lady what the object of my footrule could be; and I really dared not to ask my worthy missionary host to interpret for me." Galton projects his own particular brand of ocular desire when he notes that "the object of my admiration stood under a tree, and was turning herself about to all points of the compass, as ladies who wish to be admired usually do." His solution was to employ his sextant and take "a series of observations upon her figure in every direction, up and down, crossways, diagonally, and so forth, and I registered them carefully upon an outline drawing for fear of any mistake: this being done, I boldly pulled out my measuring tape, and measured the distance from where I was to the place where she stood, and having thus obtained both base and angles, I worked out the results by trigonometry and logarithms."[16] "Boldly pulled out" indeed, but we should duly note that what Galton pulled out was his tool of greatest desire, a tape measure, since measurement has become in this episode an activity of erotic foreplay.

We probably want to laugh at this exertion on Galton's part, but behind the risibility is a wonderful example of the confluence of the obsessive desires that drove a good deal of the engine of progress in the nineteenth century. The male gaze links up nicely with the colonial gaze and is then processed by the scientific compulsion to map, analyze, possess, and process. The id is nicely converted to the socially acceptable ego, and the impulsive reflex gives way to the obsessive-compulsive action in the ser-

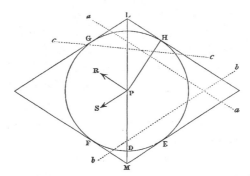

FIGURE 5. Francis Galton's diagram from *The Art of Travel* (1862).

vice of civilization. From these obsessive tics comes a wealth of "knowledge." We might suppose that the recourse to remote measurement was preferable to the kind of physical prodding and poking that the real Hottentot Venus, Saartjie Baartman, experienced when she was exhibited in London, where one observer noted that "one pinched her, another walked round her, one gentleman poked her with his cane; and one lady employed a parasol to ascertain that all was, as she called it, 'nattral.'"[17]

That Galton should have recourse to measurement in Africa is nowhere more dramatically illustrated than in his fascinating book *The Art of Travel,* which explains how to fit up a safari and travel through unchartered areas. Based on his extensive travels through Africa, the book includes mathematical formulas for finding one's way when lost, including the formula PL = PH/cos HPL = PD/cos ½ RPS and figures like that in figure 5. It's hard to imagine having the presence of mind to use such a diagram when lost in the jungle. These instructions might be somewhat daunting to a less compulsive traveler. Galton's interaction with the colonial subject did not confine itself to measuring, and the nature of the other kinds of relations tells us a bit more about the desire to measure.

Galton became a member of the Kew Observatory and subsequently its head. There he established means for standardizing sextants and other angular instruments, testing the accuracy of thermometers (providing a seal of approval for upward of twenty thousand per year), testing the performance of telescopes and opera glasses supplied to the army and navy, creating and distributing daily weather charts to newspapers. In short, the tic of measuring and analyzing became a way of standardizing what had been somewhat ineffable previously.

GENIUS AND MADNESS

Science was not simply obsessive owing to its notion of focus. There was literally an addictive side to science. Galton, while a medical student, experimented with drugs, but he was not the first. A good example of the collective addictiveness of science was to be found in the London Askesian Society, which devoted itself to scientific experiments. In January 1800 William H. Pepys used a laboratory on Plough Street to manufacture nitrous oxide, better known as laughing gas, and distributed it to members of the society. As one member, William Allen, noted, the drug had "a remarkably inebriating effect."[18] The society tried the drug several times, and Humphry Davy wrote about the gas in a series of publications, meanwhile developing a serious addiction, as did William Allen.[19]

We tend to think of science in opposition to obsession and madness, but it is also clear that for some "scientists" the pressures of the obsessive observations and other stressors of this way of life lead to psychic pain. William Allen, mentioned above, may have become addicted to various substances because of this kind of stress. Indeed his personal diaries record his daily links between the demands of being a scientist and his mental security:

> 3 December 1801: At seven o'clock I gave my first lecture on chemistry. I got through beyond my expectations, but I was very low about it before I began.
> 13 February 1802: Rose early—getting ready for experiments at the Hospital—I felt distressingly low and anxious . . .
> 21 October 1802: First lecture at the Hospital this season . . . I am very anxious and fearful.[20]

Allen's anxiety and fears, along with his addictions, were perhaps not uncharacteristic of scientists and thinkers in the nineteenth century. Many famous people during this time experienced breakdowns, including Harriet Martineau, Samuel Coleridge, Thomas Carlyle, John Stuart Mill, Matthew Arnold, Edward Bulwer-Lytton, Florence Nightingale, William James, and John Ruskin. Mill wrote about his breakdown, as did Carlyle, Arnold, Bulwer-Lytton, and James. It almost seems as if an autobiography written during the nineteenth century were required to include a section on mental breakdown, as Francis Galton's did. Mill mentions specifically that "analysis" had triggered his breakdown. Because his education, conducted largely by his strict father, had favored analysis, "my education, I thought had failed to create these feelings in sufficient strength to resist the dissolving influence of analysis, while the whole course of intellectual cultivation had made precocious and premature analysis the inveterate habit of my mind."[21] Too much study and thought had produced the societally recognized result—depression and breakdown. Mill mentions that he is not alone and remarks that "many others have passed through a similar state."[22]

Indeed, the French alienists developed systems specifically to describe mental illness that were, in part, based on notions of the link between genius and madness. The best-known proponent of this idea was Jacques Joseph Moreau, who in 1859 wrote *Morbid Psychology,* in which he stressed the continuity between various mental states by drawing a "tree of nervosity" in which the branch of "exceptional intelligence" extends next to the branch of "lesions of the central nervous system" and just above "neuroses." The branch of "exceptional intelligence" produces foliage of the "sciences" and "letters" and sprouts out another branch of "arts," with "music" and "painting" as leaves. As Moreau writes, the madman and the genius are all "born and developed under the same influence, like the effects of the same cause, like branches growing from the same tree."[23] He adds "the virtue and vices [of excessive nervous mental energy] can come from the same foyer, the virtue being the genius, the vice, idiocy."[24]

The formula is always the same. Overwork and troubles lead to a mental breakdown. Geniuses suffer more than does the common man. The philosopher Arthur Schopenhauer, writing in 1844, noted the difficulty of paying close attention to things for very long:

> Even the intellect itself is not capable of sticking very long and continuously to one idea. On the contrary, just as the eye, when it gazes for a long time at one object, is soon not able to see it distinctly any longer . . . so also through long-continued rumination on one thing our thinking gradually becomes confused and dull, and ends in a complete stupor.[25]

ATTENTION-SURFEIT DISORDER: WILKIE COLLINS'S *HEART AND SCIENCE*

On the question of this kind of sustained attention, the general understanding of the period is that such obsessive activities will inevitably lead to overwork, fatigue, and eventually madness unless the proper steps are taken. Writing in 1889, Théodule Ribot noted, "Attention is a state that is fixed. If it is prolonged beyond a reasonable time . . . everybody knows from individual experience, that there results a constantly increasing cloudiness of the mind, finally a kind of intellectual vacuity, frequently accompanied by vertigo."[26] Both Schopenhauer and Ribot, writing in roughly the same period, are interested in or concerned with this general phenomenon of excessive focus or attention. Their conclusion is consonant with many general cultural observations concerning the dangers of fixed observation, attention, or study.

Many novels of the period have characters that are overworked in this way. One might notice Dr. Ovid Vere in Wilkie Collins's 1883 novel, *Heart and Science*. Vere, who "worked as few surgeons work," is described as having "received a warning, familiar to the busy men of our time — the warning from overwrought Nature, which counsels rest after excessive work."[27] He is described as having "that morbid sensitiveness, which was one of the most serious signs of his failing health" and as having "shattered nerves [that] unmanned him" (108). Vere, relatively young, is forced to take a lengthy sea voyage (notably not a train trip, which could cause neurasthenia), and his absence causes the plot events of the novel to evolve. Collins sets up an evil nemesis named Dr. Benjulia, who specializes in "brains and nerves." Benjulia is described as having "sacrificed his professional interests to his mania for experiments in chemistry," by which Collins means the dark arts of animal vivisection and experimentation — particularly on dogs and monkeys (97). The contrast the book sets up is between the young, idealistic doctor who has overworked himself but knows that he must take a rest cure, and the older, monomaniacal researcher who has failed to see that he has become a maniac through overwork. Benjulia tells Ovid, "Your nervous system's in a nasty state. . . . You had better take care of yourself" (102). Meanwhile, Benjulia acknowledges the standard problem for the scientist: "I labour at it all day. I think of it, I dream of it, all night. It will kill me. Strong as I am, it will kill me. What do you say? Am I working myself into my grave, in the medical interests of humanity?" (190). Notably, it is knowledge and research that are the cause of Dr. Benjulia's disease. He is seen as "working incessantly — never leaving his laboratory; eating at his dreadful table; snatching an hour's rest occasionally on the floor" (211). His quest for specialized knowledge of the brain, the very activity that we have seen as characteristic of this age, is the thing that leads to his own brain disease. As Benjulia puts it, "Knowledge for its own sake is the one god I worship" (190). His own scientific experiments, using animal subjects, cause his nerves to be strained, but his activities must be carried out.

> My last experiments on a monkey horrified me. His cries of suffering, his gestures of entreaty, were like the gestures of a child. I would have given the world to put him out of his misery. But I went on. In the glorious cause I went on. My hands turned cold—my heart ached—I thought of a child I sometimes play with—I suffered—I resisted—I went on. All for Knowledge! All for Knowledge! (191)

Despite this work's obvious antivivisectionist message, Collins is clearly telling us that science, particularly as it is practiced in the nineteenth century, is a kind of mass obsession.

The other evil character in the book is Ovid's mother, Mrs. Gallilee, who is a well-respected scientist. She is addressed by the narrator at one point, who says, "See the lively modern parasites that infest Science" (286). She too, like all the major characters in the novel, has a kind of nervous breakdown as a result of overwork, fixation, or stress, and she ends up in a private asylum.

Interestingly, Collins describes his own writing of *Heart and Science* in very much these terms. In a letter to a friend, he notes, "For six months—while I was writing furiously, without cessation, [I was] one part sane and three parts mad."[28] That Collins should himself seem to suffer from mental fatigue and physical problems just shows how the problematics of obsession had so clearly infiltrated the general discourse. No longer a theory or a scientific secret, obsession is something in which ordinary humans see themselves comfortably involved.

SINGLE-MINDEDNESS IN DOUBLES: DR. JEKYLL AND MR. HYDE

From Dr. Frankenstein to Captain Nemo, the line between excessive attention to single-minded study and insanity is detailed starkly as a warning. One might find it useful to turn to Robert Louis Stevenson's famous novella *The Strange Case of Dr. Jekyll and Mr. Hyde* for another classic case of science as overwork. While Galton did not deteriorate to the extent that Dr. Jekyll did, we can see that there is something in the culture drawing the connection between genius, science, and obsession. Jekyll confesses in a pre-Freudian moment to having trouble with the two sides of his personality—his studious, scholarly side and his "certain impatient gaiety of disposition."[29] We come to see that this side, his Hyde side, is one that is involved with sexual pleasure and debauchery that he treats with "an almost morbid sense of shame" (55). What is interesting is that Jekyll regards the scientist side and the sexual side as linked, rather than opposed. As he says, "I was no more myself when I laid aside restraint and plunged in shame, than when I laboured, in the eye of day, at the furtherance of knowledge or the relief of sorrow and suffering" (55). Indeed, his observation distills down to the "thorough and primitive duality of man" (55). We can say that Stevenson in 1886 was simply expressing a by-now well-established cultural fact that obsession is not confined to the mad, that sexual obsession and scientific pursuit are the dark siblings of each other. Hyde is routinely referred to as "abnormal," "deformed," "troglodytic," with "great muscular activity" combined with "great debility of constitution." in keeping with nineteenth-century notions that degeneration and deformity were linked and themselves linked to mental illness. Hyde is described on several occasions as being a "madman" or suffering from "a cerebral disease" (51). And although Jekyll is seen as quite sane, indeed the opposite of Hyde, he is described by a fellow physician, Dr. Lanyon, as someone who "began to go wrong, wrong in the mind." His resulting work is seen as "unscientific balderdash" (12). The novel in effect dramatizes both the split between the rational and the irrational as well as the underlying connection between the obsession of science and the emergent science of obsession.

FOUCAULT AND MADNESS

It has been common since the birth-of-the-asylum discussions and the work of Foucault to think of the asylum as the liminal point in which the mad were divided off from the sane. With the beginning of a hegemony of normality, we might simply apply that notion of the establishment of a firm, secure dividing line and examine how the asylum is part of the process that closes off deviancy from bourgeois, domestic security. But that would be a mistake. Rather, as I believe I have begun to show, a different process was in order. The infiltration of partial/obsessive madness along with the idea of curability into the mainstream definition of being human in effect changed the calculus by which the concept of insanity had been formulated. The notion that obsession led to madness, that thinking on a single thing could produce monomania, that the human mind was made up of faculties that could and probably would be out of kilter, led to a humanizing of the insane and an insanizing of the human. The first step of this process was the establishment of fashionable madness, noting that partial madness was the consumer privilege of the elite of society. The French Revolution led directly to the redistributing of this franchise on elite madness to the lower classes. The poor and indigent mad people were now to be treated humanely and cured in the asylum. A flow of people into and out of the asylum, at least initially, indicated that these institutions were indeed to be considered literally as rest homes — asylums in the best sense of the word. Under Pinel's watch, La Salpêtrière's records indicate that one out of two female patients left within a year after arriving.[30] So much for the warehousing of the mad. Andrew Scull notes that Foucault's notion of the Great Confinement rested on very slim research:

> But the notion of a Europe-wide Great Confinement in these years is purely mythical. Such massive incarceration simply never occurred in England in the seventeenth and eighteenth centuries, whether one focuses one's attention on the mad, who were still mostly left at large, or on the broader category of the poor, the idle and the morally disreputable. And as Gladys Swain and Marcel Gauchet argue in *Madness and Democracy* . . . even for France, Foucault's claims about the confinement of the mad in the classical age are grossly exaggerated, if not fanciful — far fewer than 5,000 were locked up even at the end of the eighteenth century, a "tiny minority of the mad who were still scattered throughout the interior of society."[31]

But the corollary was that asylums existed because partial/obsessive madness had in effect become the rule in society. No longer was it deemed necessary to keep the mad person behind bars; now that person was to be found everywhere — in the home, the workplace, and even in the supervising office of the asylum. To be obsessive was to be human.

MADNESS AS NORMAL

This collective redefinition did not simply humanize madness; it created a bell-curve of behavior. Madness was not abnormal, but part of a range of normality. Indeed, the foundation of medicine in the nineteenth century was based to a degree on the idea of a range and balance as a description of disease. As Georges Canguilhem wrote in *The Normal and the Pathological,* this was the era that moved to a notion of disease as either too much or too little of certain states. This model is easily adapted to the mind, which is spoken of as being in or out of balance. Neurasthenia is the condition of the nerves having too little energy. Mental activity is good as long as it isn't done too much. As we saw with Galton and others, obsessive behaviors that could lead to madness could at the same time lead to science. Balance and degree become the criteria of health.

As Jennifer Fleissner observes, the rise of naturalism in literature could easily be tied to the acceptance of this new form of obsessive compulsiveness. In her reading, women's lives, particularly as described in naturalist fiction, were defined by "ongoing, nonlinear, repetitive motion—back and forth, around and around, on and on—that has the distinctive effect of seeming also like a stuckness in place . . . the repetitively compulsive everyday actions."[32] She thus suggests that the shape and form of naturalist fiction is actually more defined by this new kind of obsession and compulsion than it might seem. Thinking of Pierre Janet's work on obsession and Ribot's on "maladie du volunté," Fleissner sees the plight of the typical naturalist or modernist protagonist as part of an arc of storytelling. Entire texts, she notes, "appear stalled in their narrative trajectory by their 'compulsion to describe.'"[33] Likewise for the internal monologues in their heads, which end up defining a new type of narrative. This ruminative circling around the idea, this fixed focus of observation and description, could well describe the modernist aesthetic.

Yet women and housewives were not the only subjects on whom the obsessive-compulsive vision fell. Charles Turner Thackrah observed in 1832 that many men in British society were afflicted. He notes that merchants, master manufacturers, and practitioners of medicine and surgery were subject to "anxiety of mind." As he writes of trade and commerce, "Excessive application and anxiety, by disordering the animal economy, weaken the mental powers." And physicians were not exempt from these stresses. Thackrah notes in what is by now a familiar refrain, "The application of mind to study and research tends to impair it. Night-calls are generally thought to be very injurious."[34]

In America, after midcentury, a vision emerged in the work S. Weir Mitchell. In a series of lectures, Mitchell addressed what he saw as the "nervous temperament" or "general nervousness." He describes a group, claiming that "some of them are more or less neurasthenic people, easily tired in brain or body; but others without this, or with this peculiarity but slightly developed, are merely tremulous, nervous folks, easily agitated, over sensitive, emotional, and timid."[35] Increasingly, the qualities that had been seen as linked to the quartet subsequently came under the general category of nervousness, which itself was seen as a characteristic of the age.

Invalidism became a big issue in nineteenth-century bourgeois society. Mitchell describes this problem in detail:

> We meet in practice with a growing class of disorders in which change of social circumstances, love affairs, disappointments, and what the French call *vies manquées,* combine with physical accidents to create invalids, who united neurasthenic states with a bewildering list of hysterical phenomena. These are the "bed cases," the broken-down and exhausted women, the pests of many households, who constitute the despair of physicians, and who furnish those annoying examples of despotic selfishness, which wreck the constitutions of nurses and devoted relatives, and in unconscious or half-conscious self-indulgence destroy the comfort of every one about them.[36]

There is not space or time enough in this study to sufficiently treat invalidism,[37] but the point is that much of invalidism was seen as caused by the very factors we are discussing—overwork, obsessive focus, and so on. Indeed, the history of fatigue and what is now called "stress" is parallel to this one.[38]

By the beginning of the twentieth century, nerves were part of society. As one self-help book put it in 1911:

> One of the most striking features of society in the beginning of the twentieth century, as in the last two or three decades of the nineteenth, is the prevalence of nervous affections amongst its units. So much so is this the case that the unpleasant ailment we know as "disordered nerves" has been variously described as the "disease of the century," a "national ailment," or the "fashionable illness," by writers who have been impressed by the part played in the everyday life of the time by the waywardness of our nervous systems.[39]

The age of nervousness is also an age of degeneration, as the racialized concerns about the fitness of nations combined with notions of how the nervous system works. Capitalism, urbanization, the growth of journalism, amusements, and communication contribute to the fact that "at the present time we are one of the most neurotic and excitable races on the face of the earth" (4).

And what constitutes these nervous persons who are characteristic of their age? Physically nervous persons are "thin and delicately formed . . . quick and intelligent beyond their fellows." But the most important characteristic is that "these nervous people think a great deal too much about themselves and so increase their natural sensitiveness" (8). We again return to the notion that thinking too much, in this case about oneself, is the symptom and cause of mental distress. Obsessive concern for oneself and one's own thought processes now seems to be the key to the new citizen of the twentieth century. Indeed, "as might be expected, on the whole one finds most instances of nerve-trouble among the brain workers, and consequently it is from the better-educated sections of society in the larger cities and towns that most nerve-patients come" (47).

We have considered the connection between science, specialization, overwork, and obsession, and see that each is the other in the nineteenth century. The ensuing chapters will consider some particular manifestations of this conjunction in the areas of writing, analysis, art, and sexuality— ultimately leading us back to the contemporary vision of OCD.

4

Never Done: Compulsive Writing, Graphomania, Bibliomania

Much has been written about the nineteenth-century novel, but one characteristic has been overlooked, perhaps because it is so obvious. The great novelists of that century were engaged in a single-minded work project that had no precedent — the continuous, cumulative production of words. Dickens, Balzac, Trollope, Zola, Goncourt, and many less well-known writers have an output, an opus, that is staggering and awe-inspiring. These writers wrote not only novels but journalism, criticism, and letters — they were in effect writing all the time. They had become obsessives in the cause of letters.

NO DAY WITHOUT A SENTENCE

Of course, this isn't to say that earlier writers didn't devote themselves to writing. We have the output of Shakespeare, Milton, Defoe, Addison, Steele, and so on. But a quick survey of library shelves will make it obvious that few if any eighteenth-century (or previous) writers occupy as much shelf space as the nineteenth-century writers. Continuing projects, like those of Balzac and Zola, aimed to create a virtual world built by many volumes filled with continuing characters — Balzac's *Comédie Humaine* and Zola's Rougon-Macquart series.

The novel as a form had become the mass-produced cultural item of its time. Zola had noted that novels "multiply with terrifying fecundity. . . . Booksellers tell me that their display windows could not contain them all."[1] And the novel had become the cabinet of knowledge that claims to contain all forms of knowing. As Zola wrote, the novel, "has monopolized all space, absorbed all genres. . . . It is what one wishes it to be—a poem, a treatise on pathology, . . . a political weapon, a moral essay. One understands why most authors have adopted this eminently seductive form."[2] The form is seductive not just in its broad sweep, but in the very manner of its composition, which necessitates a kind of obsessive devotion to work. It is this period, too, that produced a concomitant obsession of reception. Readers had to read all these works and had to develop an interest in continuous reading. Very late in the nineteenth century, we find the first published interviews of authors, which created the space for fans, obsessive readership, and, of course, further production. Likewise, departments of national literature in universities began to be created, as well as chairs to study those indigenous literatures. The obsessive circle was established—voracious writing; avid reading; detailed, compulsive scholarship.

In order to produce such a volume of writing, these authors had to develop consistent and regular habits that led to daily writing in a way that fits into the general trend of monomaniacal working habits we have come to see as characteristic of the age. Indeed, Zola had inscribed on his mantelpiece the Latin phrase *nulla dies sine linea,* "no day without a sentence." Like the members of the proletariat who exchanged older desultory models of work, based on seasons, with many intervening feast days, Fat Mondays, and so on, for the efficient, repetitive work of the factory, so did writers, who had previously written when the muse struck them, or when their purses needed replenishment, who now engaged in a kind of marathon writing that often outpaced any specific monetary or even inspirational need. The case of Anthony Trollope's mother Frances was not unusual. From the age of fifty until seventy-six, she wrote 114 novels.[3] Trollope himself wrote a mere 47 novels and 16 books on other subjects. Sir Walter Scott authored over 60 works. Balzac was an obsessive collector and an obsessive writer who often sat at his desk from fifteen to eighteen hours a day, ultimately inventing over 3,000 characters.[4] Freud wrote over 150 books and articles as well as 20,000 letters.

Bulwer-Lytton, who had a breakdown as a result of writing too much, explained the standard series of disruptions that led to his nervous condition. He cites the social conditions in which children and laborers are told to "read, and read, and read."[5] Such overwork of the mind leaves the nerves "jaded and prostrate" (16). He likens the mind to a post-horse who gets no rest, until "we begin to feel the frame break under us." Drugs provide temporary relief, but eventually people are "thoroughly shattered, with complaints grown chronic, diseases fastening to the organs" (16). Bulwer-Lytton described himself as a "workman." "I began to write and to toil" when just a child. He devoted himself to writing and study so that "the wear and tear went on without intermission—the whirl of the wheel never ceased." Like Ovid Vere and others, he was advised to go on trips, which he did, but the trips made him more aware of his own infirmities so that "he had no resource but to fly from myself—to fly into the other world of books" (17). Like other nineteenth-century writers, he needed to be an obsessive worker because "as long as I was always at work it seemed that I had no leisure to be ill"(18).

CASE HISTORY OF AN OBSESSIVE: ÉMILE ZOLA

Characteristic of this kind of compulsive writer was Émile Zola, the French novelist, journalist, and social critic who wrote thirty-seven novels, ten critical works, and countless pieces of journalism, art criticism, and letters.[6]

Zola was perhaps the first (if not only) writer to allow himself not only to be interviewed and scrutinized but also to become the object of scientific and medical study. His level of output and force of personality were so extraordinary that he was considered worthy of detailed scientific observation by a team of researchers. In keeping with contemporary notions of eugenics and statistics, every part of Zola's body and mind, including his writing habits, was examined and calibrated as if he were an oddity or monstrosity, as, in some sense, he was. Arthur MacDonald, the author of a book called *Abnormal Man,* wrote in 1898 two articles in which he reviewed the findings of this study of Zola for American readers. As Mac-Donald put it, the study undertaken by over fifteen scientists was "the most thorough one ever made of an individual in society (a number have been made on criminals in prison)."[7]

One of the reasons, no doubt, that Zola allowed this massive scientific undertaking was that his own theory of art was devoted to the notion that the novel, as a form, was a kind of scientific experiment that could in effect provide a controlled study of the lives of his characters based on hereditary traits and the influence of environment. Indeed, his entire Rougon-Macquart series follows the fate of two founding families as their inherited traits interact with their social milieu. As Zola wrote in the introduction to the second edition of *Thérèse Raquin,* "Scientific truth was my touchstone for every scene. . . . He who reads the novel with care will see that each chapter explores a curious physiological phenomenon."[8] In preparation for his project, he did research at the Bibliothèque Impériale, consulting works by Bernard, Morel, Letourneau, Moreau de Tours, and Lucas on madness, degeneration, and heredity physiology.[9] Indeed, in a brief memorandum entitled "Differences between Balzac and Me," he wrote, "My work will be less social than scientific. . . . It is especially important that I remain a naturalist, a physiologist. . . . It will suffice to be a scientist, to describe what is by searching for what lies underneath. No conclusion, moreover. A simple exposé of the facts of a family showing the inner mechanism that makes it run."[10] As Zola wrote in *The Experimental Novel,* "It is scientific investigation, it is experimental reasoning, which combats one by one the hypotheses of the idealists, and which replaces purely imaginary novels by novels of observation and experimentation."[11] Zola's admiration of science, and his belief that science, as the functioning arm of a democratic, nontheological state, would set the world free was key to his own writing and to his willingness to be observed in detail by physiologists and alienists. Indeed, probably more than any other nineteenth-century writer, Zola deeply believed in the scientific explanations of madness as it was explicated through hereditary arguments and notions of degeneracy. His own work is a virtual catalog of obsessions and compulsions running through families, particularly focusing on the major areas of obsession—sex, murder, work, and art.

But science, as we have seen and will see, is itself an obsessive activity that involves various possible manias. We want to keep in mind that someone like Zola is both subject and object to such minds. His work is defined as science, and his being is subject to science. Thus Zola agreed not only to be studied by a committee of doctors, but also to have the study published. The translation from the physical body to the body in words was a natural one for him. "I have read these pages [of the study], they have interested me much, and I willingly grant authority to publish them as authentic and true; for I have one desire in life, the truth, and one purpose, to make the most of truth."[12] Zola notes that "in the thousands of pages I have written, I have nothing to withdraw. . . . The study of me is about one who has given his life to work and dedicated to this work all his physical, mental, and moral forces."[13] Zola equates himself with his own words, his production of words, which are equivalent, in some sense, to his physical body and his mental state. In this sense, physical analysis by doctors and literary analysis by critics are all the same thing, as is his own "scientific" study that is embodied in his literary work. Indeed, Zola compiled huge dossiers on the subject and plotting of each novel before he wrote it, and he consciously decided to donate his dossiers to the public, along with his complete correspondence, for the reason, we must assume, that such information would add to the science of writing about his own work as production.[14]

This circle from science to work, work to body, body to mind, and then back to science is part of the obsessional structure of the nineteenth century. A significant part of science involves the single-minded study of humans, and, in turn, being human in modern life is becoming single-minded and obsessive in relation to life, work, and sexuality. It is for this reason that the case study, soon to become the "truest" way of knowing a person, will find its fulfillment in the work of Freud and Josef Breuer, having been previously developed in the laboratory of the novel.[15]

The case study of Zola at fifty-seven begins with his early years, in which his illnesses, including a violent fever, "probably cerebral," are described. The onset of puberty "was characterized by a certain timidity, as is often the case with neuropathic persons on account of inhibitory ideas."[16] By the time he reached early adulthood, he was described as living a life of "material privations." These, connected with his "intense intellectual activity," combined with his "congenital neurotic condition" to produce his "nervous troubles" (469). The symptoms of his nervous troubles were intestinal pains between the ages of twenty and forty; from forty-five to fifty, cystitis and angina. He also had "morbid ideas" and "gastric dilation, pyrosis, stomachal pains, and drowsiness after eating"(469).

The study then goes on to very detailed biometrics measuring his proportions, taking his hand and fingerprints, his respiration, pulse, hand strength, and so on. There is a particular fascination with the dynamometer, which measures hand strength, a measure of overall fitness. Zola shows signs of weakening after writing for an hour, particularly after writing for three hours. While this pseudoscience is amusing, it is also cautionary in its reliance on "objective" measurements—bodily data—which are then interpreted as the scientist sees fit. The attempt is to correlate the physical symptom with the mental disorder. The logic could then be used to work backward from mental disorder to physical degeneracy. Max Nordau, who judged Zola to be a degenerate author, said that science could bypass the biometrics and go straight to the mental disorder. Thus, "it is not necessary to measure the cranium of an author, or to see the lobe of a painter's ear, in order to recognize the fact that he belongs to the class of degenerates."[17] Nordau's solution was simply to look at the work and then infer the nervous conditions. He notes various diagnostic names given to authors, including "higher degenerates" and more tellingly "graphomaniacs" or "semi-insane persons who feel a strong impulse to write."[18] This definition turns out to be a fairly good one for many nineteenth-century authors.

As an example of the scientific interest in finding physical correlates to mental conditions and vice versa, the section on Zola's nervous system is telling:

> Zola's nervous system in its entirety presents cardiac spasms, cramps, pollakiuria, trembling, etc. It is notably subject to crises of pain, which date from the age of twenty. From this time on to forty there were periods of nervous colic. From forty-five to fifty these crises took the form of angina pectoris, of acute cystitis, and of articular rheumatisms. At present these troubles are less, but they are replaced by a state of almost constant feebleness and irritability. Sometimes gastric troubles are the occasion of nervous manifestations, but at present it is intellectual or muscular effort which provokes them; sometimes the slightest thing is sufficient to awake them, such as a too close fitting garment; thus the squeezing in a crowd once provoked a crisis of agony with false angina pectoris; so the pricking of a finger has been felt in his arm for several hours.[19]

The conclusion is that Zola displays "a lack of nervous equilibrium," which is to say that his nervous system is out of balance. And of course, the cause is "intellectual superiority," which is caused itself by "exercise of brain and mind" (478). As we have seen consistently, the devotion to doing one thing too much, the overdevelopment of intellectual faculties particularly, is seen as the dominant cause of nervous problems.

It is in this moment that we begin to see the developing contradiction of obsession as a social and cultural category. On the one hand, a single-minded devotion to an idea must be a good thing, and certainly is a sign of human progress. On the other, it is seen as a problem that leads to degeneration of the human species. The scientists who observe Zola are faced with this problem—is Zola a man of genius or a degenerate? In the study of Zola, one of the features noted was his ability in "distinguishing odors [in which] he shows the finest precision. . . . His memory of olfactory sensations is very strong. Odors play a prominent role in his writings as well as his life" (479). Yet Max Nordau had critiqued degenerate fiction, particularly the work of Zola, as being characterized by exactly this point—an overconcern for odors. Nordau cites as authority the work of Leopold Bernard, whose book *Les odeurs dans le roman de Zola* published in 1889, collects in a somewhat obsessive way all the passages in Zola's novels that touch on smells. Nordau concludes that Zola is an author with "an unhealthy predominance of the sensations of smell in his consciousness, and a perversion of the olfactory which makes the worst odours, especially those of all human excretions, appear to him particularly agreeable and sensually stimulating."[20]

Indeed, the battle for the team of doctors was to define Zola without consigning him to the refuse heap of degeneration. One can feel the analytic method, which almost by necessity turns the observed subject into a medicalized malformation, in conflict with the realization that the subject of study isn't just any patient but a world-historical writer. The conclusion made by Édouard Toulouse, Zola's personal physician, that "he has never seen an obsessed or impulsive person who was so well balanced"[21] sounds like the punch line to a Woody Allen joke. But the import of this statement is that it tries to reconcile the notion of obsession in artistic modes with a notion of normalcy in the context of a bioculturally understood form of modernity. One can see this tension in the statement "Although he [Zola] has many nervous troubles, the term 'degeneracy' does not apply to him wholly" (484). The point is that while Zola is a degenerate, he isn't wholly one. Strangely, the next sentence then points in the other direction. "Magnan classes him among those degenerates who, though possessing brilliant faculties, have more or less mental defects" (484).[22] MacDonald goes on to parse out this contradiction: "It is true, as we have seen, that Zola has orbicular contraction, cardiac spasms, thoracic cramps, false angina pectoris, sensory hyperaesthesia, obsessions, and impulsive ideas; his emotivity is defective, and certain of his ideas are morbid, but all this is not sufficient to affect in any appreciable manner his intellectual processes (484)." Again, there is certain retrospective humor to the effect of watching a paradigm twist in its own contradiction. You almost expect him to add "but no one's perfect."

The report refers to a specific kind of obsession focused on the "tendency for order" which is "so strong that it sometimes reaches a morbid stage, for it provokes a certain suffering in cases of disorder" (484). Zola is described as having various manias, particularly the by now well-known "doubting mania." This centered on fears of "not being able to do his daily task; or of being incapable of completing a book."[23] Another was "arithmetical mania," in which he counted gas jets on the street, the number of doors, taxis, steps, objects on his bureau. He also had to touch the same pieces of furniture a certain number of times before going to sleep. He felt it was necessary to open his eyes seven times at night to prevent his dying. Certain numbers were ominous, and these numbers changed daily. So, for example, he would not hire a taxi if the license numbers added up to a "bad" number. Modern readers will recognize that these are some features of obsessive-compulsive disorder.[24]

It is also interesting to recall that some of these activities, particularly counting things and touching objects, were also described as characteristics of Dr. Samuel Johnson, although the tone and attitude in the eighteenth century toward such eccentricities were very different.[25] What we are seeing is the attempt to develop a purely "scientific" discourse in relation to the human body and its activities. But the text we are considering is also clearly torn between the authority of the case history and the particularity of the human being so described.

MacDonald concludes that "Zola is a neuropath, that is, a man whose nervous system is painful." In the parlance of the time, there is something wrong with Zola's nervous system, that entire system that controls the organs and that regulates sensations. Zola's is not in good balance and is too susceptible to painful sensations. MacDonald assumes that "heredity seems to have caused this tendency," by which he means that Zola is disposed to this condition by the attributes passed along by his parents. However, that predisposition is activated because "constant intellectual work affected the health of his nervous tissues."[26]

Again, there is a tension between the obvious benefit of working hard at writing books and the dangers to oneself, particularly if there is a hereditary predisposition involved. This might be considered an earlier version of Freud's dilemma in *Civilization and Its Discontents,* which wonders about the split between instinctual life and the strictures of modernity. But MacDonald's dilemma is more the reverse; what if one's instincts drive one to write excessively, to focus to closely on a specialization, while the mind resists and produces symptoms? "Now, it is a question whether this neuropathical condition is not an excitation that has given rise to the intellectual ability of Zola. Whether a diseased nervous system is a necessary cause of great talent or genius."[27] MacDonald raises one of the central questions of the era—is disease the necessary condition of genius and modernity? Is what it means to be modern a kind of fixed and focused attention and awareness that has to be considered, from a theoretical point of view, pathological? Is Zola a genius or a graphomaniac? Or both?

The dossier on Zola, both as a document and as a sign of the times, raises the issue of the pathological nature of writing—of obsessive writing, writing done on a regular, daily basis to the exclusion of much else. We might also see that kind of writing as the more or less normal state of any author today. One of the features of modernity, it would seem, is the naturalization of the pathology of writing.

ZOLA'S *THE MASTERPIECE* AS AN EXPLORATION OF OBSESSION

Zola well recognized that what he did as a writer was perhaps strange and obsessive. His motto, "No day without a sentence," suggests to us the seriousness of his project. His own work discusses the issue of obsessively working at such projects, most notably his sketch for *La Rêve,* in which he envisioned "a man of forty, hitherto engrossed in science, who never having loved, now falls passionately in love with a child of sixteen." He added telegraphically, "Me; work; literature, which has consumed my life."[28] Zola's friend Edmond de Goncourt recounts a conversation with Zola in which Goncourt had been noting "the way we had given our lives to letters, given them as lives had perhaps never been given in any previous age, and we admitted to each other that we had been true martyrs of literature and maybe even damned fools." Zola then replied, "As my wife isn't here I can tell you that I can't see a young woman like that one over there walk by without thinking: Isn't that worth more than a book?"[29] Zola's recourse to compare life, as embodied in a young woman, with the staggering compilation of words that amounts to his oeuvre leads to a conclusion that his way of life, the life of genius and of writing, may be a kind of sinkhole of human energy and a distraction from something more palpable. This is, always, the dilemma of any obsession—is it anything or is it nothing? Zola could not figure out, in this regard, if "I am the laziest man in the world or the most industrious" (616). His writing four pages a day, year after year, had brought him to a "crisis," like so many writers in the nineteenth century. As he engages in "constant swotting" to finish the last of the Rougon-Macquart series, he notes that he is "cloistered . . . from morning 'til night" without seeing anyone (617). While this kind of isolation may indeed be the rule for writers, Zola pinpoints it as a cause for illness in his novel *L'oeuvre* (*The Masterpiece*).

Zola's obsessive work shows up in the double-entendre title of this novel, in which Claude Lantier devotes his life to the *work* of painting a *masterpiece* so that the work, both masterpiece and life activity, consume him utterly. His typical day involves "spurning meat and drink, working like a madman in an endless struggle with nature."[30]

He "lived only for his picture," which was "the sole aim and end of his existence" (265, 269). Claude wonders, "Wouldn't it be wonderful to devote one's whole life to one work . . . ?" (43). Tellingly, his project, as was Zola's own, was to show "modern life in all its aspects, that's the subject" (44). Modernity is embodied in the specific work and in the general work—both of which are an obsession and obsessive. Claude is not the only obsessive in this regard; Christine, his mistress then wife, is also focused on Claude's masterpiece, but from a different direction. The painting becomes a hysterical symptom of the couple's monofocus. Christine's relation to Claude is "an idée fixe" and the painting steals his attention from her, as the living model, to the two-dimensional nude in the painting (96). Claude is "obsessed" (121) initially by the image of Christine's youthful body, but quickly shifts from her body to the figure of the woman he is painting, an object that becomes "the fixed idée they shared in silence" (122). To be the nude model for the painting again becomes "an overwhelming obsession" to her, but to Claude the real woman will never be equal to the painting in which he "found in his art, the everlasting pursuit of unattainable beauty, the mad desire which could never be satisfied" (275, 280). That this fixation is pathological is signaled in plot logic by the birth of their child, who has "an enormous head which marked him as the blemished offspring of genius" (251).

As Claude degenerates under the weight of his obsession, he begins to have the kind of symptomatology that Zola himself had. Zola uses the language of psychology and neurology when he describes Claude's hypochondriacal thinking about his physical problems: "Could it mean that the lesions, the imagined existence of which had caused him so much worry in the past, were increasing? As his crises recurred more and more frequently, he would spend weeks in unbearable self-torture" (236).[31] In either case, Claude's obsessions have a focal location that becomes dependent on his art and his work. Like Zola, he has various kinds of manias, such as a "mania of his to paint from right to left . . . [because] he was sure it was lucky."[32]

The oeuvre itself suffers fatally from this obsessive devotion. His drawings become frenzied, and he draws "with so much energy that he cut clean through the paper." Claude begins to add explanatory diagrams and words so that his sketches are "rapidly overloaded with endless summary details [and] soon became such an inextricable tangle of line that she [Christine] could make nothing of it all" (247). Claude's obsession with the work turns to revulsion, such that in succession he stabs his canvas, punches his fist through it, scrapes off all the paint, and finally tears it into pieces and burns it.

But the most telling section of the novel is when Sandoz, Claude's writer friend, rails against the idea of work, showing that his work as an author and Claude's as a painter are the essence of obsession. It is generally held that Claude is actually a representation of Cézanne, Zola's childhood friend, and Sandoz would then be Zola himself. I quote at length to show the frenzied and extensive way that Zola presents this obsession:

The thing is, work has simply swamped my whole existence. Slowly but surely it's robbed me of my mother, my wife, and everything that meant anything to me. It's like a germ planted in the skull that devours the brain, spreads to the trunk and limbs, and destroys the entire body in time. No sooner am I out of bed in the morning than work clamps down on me and pins me to my desk before I've even had a breath of fresh air. It follows me to lunch and I find myself chewing over sentences as I'm chewing my food. It goes with me when I go out, eats out of my plate at dinner and shares my pillow in bed at night. It's so completely merciless that once the process of creation is started, it's impossible for me to stop it, and it goes on growing and working even when I'm asleep. . . . Outside that, nothing, nobody exists. I go up to see my mother, but I'm so absorbed that ten minutes afterwards I'm asking myself whether I've been up to her or not. As for my wife, she has no husband, poor thing; . . . But do what I will, I can't escape entirely from the monster's clutches, and I'm soon back in the semiconscious state that goes with creation and just as sullen and indifferent as I always am when I'm working. . . . I haven't even a will of my own; it's become a habit now to lock my door on the world outside and throw my key out of the window. . . . So there we are, cribbed and confined together, my work and me. And in the end it'll devour me, and that will be the end of that. (302–3)

The work that Claude is engaged in, which the narrator describes as "his endless task" (359), becomes more and more incoherent and maniacal. Claude is now described openly as having an "obsession," being a "maniac in his madness," and acting "like a maniac to his mania" (400–405). Work becomes the justification for life, but work also becomes the meaningless devotion to a single-minded and increasingly narrow and disoriented endeavor. As in Zola's case, Claude can't decide whether this devotion is everything or nothing. "But how can I go on living if there's no point in going on working? . . . . The only thing that would make life worth living would be something that doesn't exist" (409).

When Claude finally succumbs and kills himself, his friends say of him, "He'd a hero's capacity for work . . . yet he has nothing to show" (417). In fact, Claude's is the fate not of a single madman, but of an entire generation. One friend remarks, "We're living in a bad season, in a vitiated atmosphere, with the century coming to an end and everything in process of demolition. . . . How can anybody expect to be healthy? The nerves go to pieces, general neurosis sets in, and art begins to totter, faced with a free-for-all, with anarchy to follow" (421). This fin-de-siècle viewpoint is compounded by a psychological contradiction—to be artists in this generation is to be diseased by the very force that makes them artists in the first place. They are torn between creativity and neurosis, both of which are the hallmarks of their time. Work, which had been the simple province of the peasants, the thing that kept them sane, is now transmuted to monomaniacal labor, most notably writing, which is no longer salutary but dangerous. Most remarkably, the last line of the novel, uttered by Sandoz, whose previous diatribe against work sits hauntingly over the entire novel, is the unforgettable "And now, back to work!" (426).

We might want to take this argument a step farther. The analysis of Zola as an author/patient and the analysis of literary texts seem to be projects destined to intersect. In the opening of *Thérèse Raquin* Zola explicitly brings up the subject of analysis using language that sounds as if it is part of the medical survey of Zola himself: "I hope that by now it is becoming clear that my object has been first and foremost a scientific one. . . . I simply applied to two living bodies the analytical method that surgeons apply to corpses. . . . The writer is simply an analyst . . . who has done so as a surgeon might in an operating theater."[33] Zola's use of the terms "analyst" and "analysis" in 1867 alerts us to the French usage that allows for the term to be used in surgery and mathematics. It may well be that Freud, coming to Paris to study with Jean-Martin Charcot, picked up this usage and applied it to psychoanalysis as he did in the 1890s. In any case, what we see is the crossover from science to literature and then eventually back to science. Analysis of characters, a literary text, or the human psyche was clearly an activity whose time had come. When we consider that this kind of analysis is simply another way of talking about obsession, the studying of one thing very carefully and in focused detail, the issue of the two-faced interconnection of observer and observed comes to the fore. For Zola as for Freud, for Charcot as for Marie Bichat, the matter was analysis that revealed the fixed attention and desires of patients and characters while it disguised the position of the observer.

FOLIE À DEUX: BOUVARD AND PÉCUCHET

It would be remiss to discuss obsession and novels of this period without looking at Gustave Flaubert's signal work on the subject. *Bouvard and Pécuchet,* unfinished and perhaps unfinishable at the author's death, is a cross between a novel and a philosophical rant whose topic is nothing less than a view of modernity as a world gone mad with obsessiveness. As *Caleb Williams* was the book that began the cult of obsession in literature, Flaubert's work is a kind of capstone to the arc of monomania, idée fixe, and scientific study.

The opening of *Bouvard and Pécuchet* invokes the world of monotonous work that one recognizes now as one of the causes of neurasthenia. The two men, both copyists in offices, meet each other one day while sitting on a park bench. What draws them together is the fact that each notices that the other has written his own name on the inside of his hat. The act of labeling their headwear belongs to a world in which individuality is vying with mass culture—hats are identical, can be lost, ergo names have to be inscribed, especially in offices where people are interchangeable. This is the world of the modern neurasthenic, as described by George Beard.

Indeed, Bouvard and Pécuchet meet in one of those harsh, unattractive borderlands of modernity described by Timothy J. Clark in his book *The Painting of Modern Life,* in which the suburbs emerge from the scrubland of industry and commerce—the very place painted by the impressionists and by Claude in Zola's *The Masterpiece.* Flaubert's book recounts Bouvard and Pécuchet's comic and pathetic flight from the world of this alienated landscape to a rural retreat. But the rural retreat is no escape from the culture, because in it they reproduce obsessively an encyclopedic range of knowledges by reading though and devoting themselves to virtually all branches of the arts and sciences.

The book is not only about obsession in its modern sense, but about the world that creates that obsessive attention. It is a world influenced and suffused by science, so both men "extol the advantages of science: so many things to know, so much research . . . if only one had the time!"[34] Science, by definition, requires endless attention and study. Their project is literally to devote themselves to every aspect of science and learning by quitting their jobs and using their leisure time as work time. Ideas and facts become items to be collected; the gathering up of one thing leads to the need for other things.

"At the National Library they would have liked to know the exact number of volumes." "The more ideas they had the more they suffered" (28, 29). The world they occupy is one that requires a kind of repetition, so when they hear a new witticism it "amused them so much that twenty times a day, for more than two weeks, they repeated it" (39). Indeed, for Flaubert, modernity is characterized by the endless repetition of received ideas, so much so that he wrote a *Dictionary of Received Ideas* that lists words used over and over again in clichéd ways. For example, take this series:

> WINTER: Always "unusual." (See SUMMER) Is healthier than the other
> seasons.
> WIT: Always preceded by "sparkling.". . .
> WITNESS: Always refuse to be a witness. You never know where it may
> lead you.

The characters in the novel turn to the vast wealth of knowledge in books as their sure guide to confronting human sciences and technologies such as farming and architecture. But since their knowledge comes only from reading various authorities, the result of much of what they do lacks coherence. Flaubert himself read over 1,500 books to authenticate this novel, and the novel itself is, in its turn, a kind of massive catalog of those works and the knowledges in them. but all that reading, as we have seen to be the case in the world of overwork, "had disturbed their brains" (82). And again the sheer number of facts is overwhelming. Pécuchet despairs: "The sun is a million times bigger than the earth, Sirius twelve times bigger than the sun, comets are 34,000,000 leagues long!" And Bouvard laments, "It's enough to drive one mad!" (84). Facts drive one mad by their sheer numbers, and art drives one mad by its passions. As one doctor says to Pécuchet, "Take a purge . . . too full of nerves, too artistic!" (147).

Their pursuits become fixations. As Flaubert notes, "Diet obsessed them" (77). Among the medical scientists they study, examples of science gone obsessive abound. For example, they decide to emulate Sanctorius, who, to prove his theory that our body surface gives off a measurable vapor, "spent half a century daily weighing his food with all his excretions, and weighing himself, only taking time off to write down his calculations" (74). While their activities are selected by Flaubert for humor, he, like Swift referring to the Academy at Lagado, made sure that the experiments they did were based on actually documented ones. Even their use of "the new fashion of inserting thermometers into their rectums," which causes "great scandal," eventually becomes common practice (79). It is hard to tell what is satirized and what is science. And that is the point of a modernity in which attention and obsession become the rule. The protagonists reach a point where they depress each other with doubting and fearing everything, including what they eat and drink: "A glass of water in the morning is 'dangerous.' Every food or drink was followed by a similar warning, or by the word: 'Bad!—Be careful not to abuse it!—Does not agree with everyone!" (82). The study of diet gives way to geology, and then "obsession with the Flood gave way to an obsession with erratic blocks [of stone]" (92). Each subject area proves "defective," and finally they begin to see that the quest for certainty, which is the goal of science, is itself an obsessive activity. The desire to know and catalog is held up to a kind of ridicule by Flaubert. Indeed, in a strange prefiguration of Freud, they begin to see phallic symbols everywhere.

In former times towers, pyramids, candles, milestones and even trees had a phallic significance, and for Bouvard and Pécuchet everything became phallic. They collected swing-poles of carriages, chair-legs, cellar bolts, pharmacists' pestles. When people came to see them they would ask: "What do you think that looks like?" then confided the mystery, and if there were objections, they shrugged their shoulders pityingly. (114–15)

The obsessive vision sees coherence in all things. Such a way of seeing becomes over time the clinical gaze, the collator's or collector's vision.

Indeed, the whole project of knowing comes under Flaubert's ironic scrutiny and begins to seem itself an impossibly compulsive activity. "To judge impartially they would have had to read all the histories, all the memoirs, all the journals, and all the manuscript documents, for the slightest omission may cause an error which will lead to others ad infinitum. They gave up" (121). This view of knowledge highlights the driven inclusiveness of scholarly activity. Specialization requires uninterrupted study of an ever-expanding body of knowledge that itself must, by definition, lack coherence.

In fact, Bouvard and Pécuchet are in an endless process of giving up and then trying again, like some nineteenth-century version of the road-runner and the coyote. In one of the most preposterous, but then also aptly metaphoric, moments, Bouvard and Pécuchet realize that they cannot remember all the information about French history that they need to in order to begin to understand. So they use Dumochel's memory training system (learned, of course, from another book), which is itself mind-boggling rather than mind-training. In it numbers are replaced by mnemonic figures—so that 1 is a tower, 2 a bird, 3 a camel, and so on. Bouvard and Pécuchet use their house as the "mnemotechnic" base, "attaching to each of its parts one distinct fact, and the yard, the garden, the surroundings, the whole region no longer had any other sense than to aid memory. Boundary stones in their countryside delimited certain periods, the apple-trees were genealogical trees, bushes were battles, the whole world became a symbol" (123). In this altered reality, real things become symbolic of things that need to be remembered so that the facts of history can be recalled. But the whole project seems beyond pointless.

Finally, they begin the obsessive reading of novels, which seems to close the loop of the obsessive study of things obsessive. It is no coincidence that Flaubert himself wrote at the age of fifteen a short story called "Bibliomania" in which a bookseller is obsessed with books. "This passion entirely absorbed him. He scarcely ate, he no longer slept, but he dreamed whole days and nights of his fixed idea: books."[35] Novels, however, add another dimension of "stuckness," to use Jennifer Fleissner's term, since their plots are based on repetition and recurrence. Bouvard is bored by Walter Scott's work because of the "repetition of the same effects."[36] They turn to Balzac, who wrote about every aspect of life in France, so inevitably his work soon becomes as much of a catalog as anything else in *Bouvard and Pécuchet:* "He [Balzac] writes one novel about chemistry, another about banking, another on printing machines. . . . We'll have one on every trade and every province, then on every town and every floor of every house, and every individual, and it will not be literature, but statistics or ethnography" (133). Perhaps aiming a critique at realism, Flaubert sees novels as now so close to exposition of scientific methods, anthropology, sociology, that the literary aspect drops out. Writing becomes an endless, obsessive project.

In despair, Bouvard and Pécuchet give up their pursuits and try to live a religious life, although they manage to ask so many questions of their priest that he insists they "worship without understanding" (235). But they miss their obsessions, which gave them purpose. "Where were the days when they used to go into farms, looking everywhere for antiques? Nothing now could bring about those delightful hours filled with distilling or literature" (218). In that last line, Flaubert captures the necessity of obsession—to be modern you can't live with obsession and you can't live without it. It would take Freud to make that necessity explicit.

BIBLIOMANIA

As Flaubert notes, there is a nexus between work, writing, books, the obsessive reading of books, and the collecting of books. It is no coincidence that the late eighteenth and nineteenth centuries saw the efflorescence of bibliomania—most specifically defined as the collecting of books, involving the desire to buy, own, and store books, often disassociated from any desire to read those books. The term was first used in English by Lord Chesterfield in the eighteenth century, obviously borrowing from the French, when he advised his son to "beware of the *Bibliomanie.*"[37] But the term was first used as a disease reference in an 1809 poem by John Ferriar, a physician who supervised the "anti-mania" ward at the Manchester Lunatic Hospital. Ferriar wrote in his poem "The Bibliomania":

What wild desires, what torments seize
The hapless man who feels the book disease. . . .[38]

Although somewhat tongue-in-cheek, the work nevertheless is rooted in the emergent notion of monomania. The desire for books is called "a tyrant passion" that "drags them [the book collectors] backwards" (92). Ferriar even refers to himself in describing this disease saying:

Ev'n I, debarred of ease, and studious hours,
Confess, mid' anxious toil, its lurking pow'rs. (92)

Isaac D'Israeli wrote in 1807 that "the Bibliomania has never raged more violently than in the present age," and that the libraries of those bibliomaniacs were "madhouses of the human mind."[39] Two years later Thomas Frognall Dibdin wrote a book called *The Bibliomania*. A medical edge appears in the book's citation of the physician Ferriar's poem. We might want to recall that Dibdin had himself written a poem, "Vaccinia," now lost, that praised the scientific invention of vaccination. Dibdin was in addition a member of the Society for Scientific and Literary Disquisition, also known as "The Lunatics." So interwoven into the bibliomania fabric is a medicalized vision of madness, which Dibdin refers to as "the book disease" or "the madness of book-collecting."[40]

Dibdin goes on to describe this disease as one of males, for the most part, and specifically "people in the higher and middling ranks of society," and locates the victims as those living in "palaces, castles, halls, and gay mansions."[41] These are the very people who were the victims of the quartet, the best and brightest of British society. Dibdin enumerates the symptoms, especially the craving for black-letter editions, and the cure of the disease in the proliferation of more books, editions, and libraries so that individuals will not feel under pressure to perform the function of preservation and collection. While his book is somewhat facetious, it nevertheless captures a particular moment of obsession when mania and collecting collide.

A very good example of a bibliomaniac would be Sir Thomas Phillips, a self-described "vello-maniac," who had in nineteenth-century England the largest and most important collection of books and manuscripts ever accumulated by one person. He collected not only books but Babylonian cylinder seals, deeds, documents, genealogical charts, autograph letters, maps, and master drawings. He described himself as having "the old Mania of Book-buying."[42] His stated and capitalized goal was to "have ONE COPY OF EVERY BOOK IN THE WORLD!!!"[43] By the end of his life he had acquired over fifty thousand books and a hundred thousand manuscripts. He had amassed "more than double the size," as Henry Bradshaw wrote in 1869, "of the whole of our Cambridge University & College collections of MSS. put together."[44] A move from one residence to another required 103 wagon loads drawn by 230 horses and requiring 160 men.

With all his wealth, one would imagine that Sir Thomas would have lived in luxury, but Sir Frederic Madden, the keeper of manuscripts of the British Museum, wrote in his diary a revealing entry when he visited:

> The house looks more miserable and dilapidated every time I visit it, and there is not a room now that is not crowded with large boxes full of MSS. The state of things is really inconceivable. Lady P is absent, and were I in her place, I would never return to so wretched an abode. . . . Every room is filled with heaps of papers, MSS, books, charters, packages & other things, lying in heaps under your feet, piled upon tables, beds, chairs, ladders &c.&c. and in every room, piles of huge boxes, up to the ceiling, containing the more valuable volumes! It is quite sickening. . . . The windows of the house are never opened, and the close confined air & smell of the paper & MSS. Is almost unbearable.[45]

When Jared Sparks, the president of Harvard, was invited, Phillips warned, "The Drawing Room is the only Room we live in & 3 Bed Rooms for ourselves and our friends." Three years later he wrote that "our Drawing Room and Sitting Room is Lady Phillips' Boudoir. . . . [There] is no room to dine in except in the Housekeeper's Room!"[46]

Like Balzac's, Phillips's collecting ultimately led to profound debt. Yet the collecting continued as a profession and an avocation. This type of collecting was characteristic of the era, when the great collections were established and then found their way into museums and libraries. In a way, we would not have the major and minor works preserved in our archives were it not for the obsessive and compulsive activities of a few people. And not only did collectors collect books, but other people wrote about their obsessions. John Hill Burton's 1881 work *The Book Hunter* describes a number of such bibliomaniacs. Burton freely describes the desire to collect as a "malady" and notes of one Archdeacon Meadow, "In him truly the bibliomania may be counted among the many illustrations of the truth so often moralized on, that the highest natures are not exempt from human frailty in some shape or other."[47]

In this chapter, we've seen how obsession became so interwoven into literary and aesthetic life that it was virtually inseparable from the idea of artistic temperament or of the socially and economically defined role of the author, and that books themselves are the tokens and the substance of this obsessive behavior both in creation and consumption. Whether the object is the material book itself or the process of creating it, obsession permeates the literary sensorium. At the same time, the wellspring of creativity becomes likely to be the source of disease. The obsessed human psyche transforms into the diseased human psyche by a few twists of the conceptual dial. Given those modulations, obsession will be transmuted by psychoanalysis into one of the preeminent structuring disorders of the human mind.

5

Freud and Obsession as the Gateway to Psychoanalysis

In the history of obsession, the greatest single figure is Sigmund Freud. It has been usual to think of Freud as the heroic discoverer of the unconscious, sexual drives, and the like. But as this brief history of obsession has already shown, Freud came very late in the line of people contemplating obsession. All of the key notions that Freud dealt with were established well before him—hysteria, obsession, compulsion, mania, neurosis, transference, the unconscious, the sexual etiology of disease, and so on. It is for the convenience of our own obsessions that we have made Freud the opening act of the mental show, the moment when the curtain lifts on modern psychology.

Freud is our obsession. We live with him, use his terms, banish him, and reaccept as the times dictate. But we never stop thinking about him. He is the ruminative center of our thoughts about thoughts. He is the ur-father, the primal son, and the embodiment of the superego. Even when he's out of fashion we never stop thinking about him. We obsess that Freud invented sex—made it dirty, made it clean, made it the cause of illness and the cure of a disease. Again, this would be our own obsession, since nineteenth-century studies of mental illness gave a sexual etiology to mental illness long before Freud was even conceived by those very genital means that obsessed him. Richard von Krafft-Ebing had already written his *Psychopathia Sexualis* well before Freud began his major statements. Helen Lefkowitz Horowitz in her book *Rereading Sex* points out that four main lines of thinking, perhaps included in the ones we have been considering, contributed to the rise of a "sexual culture." These were notions based on the humoral theory, notions based around "body, nerves, health, and the relation of mind and body,"[1] Evangelical Christianity's distrust of the flesh, and various discourses which "placed sex at the center of life." It was into that latter culture that Freud was born and to which he elaborated its own ideas. In other words, for Freud to have invented an obsession with sex, the obsession with sex had to have invented him.

PSYCHOANALYSIS AS OBSESSION

We also do not have to look far for notions that sexual dysfunction led to hysteria and mental maladies. Krafft-Ebing saw the cause of neurosis as a perversion of normal, that is to say heterosexual, sexual life. The unremitting assault on masturbation was a hallmark of nineteenth-century mental hygiene.[2] Even ordinary physicians began to notice that their patients were "obsessed" with sexuality as the medical profession became equally obsessed.[3] One physician wrote in 1895, "The sexual element plays a most important part in the psychical life of woman."[4]

So Freud's emphasis on sexuality was in some sense a result rather than the cause of that obsession. Freud tells us quite clearly that the repression of childhood masturbation is the most prevalent cause of neurosis (*SE* 20: 217). In doing so, he is putting himself in line with the thinking of, if not his era (since some of his younger colleagues disagreed with this negative emphasis on masturbation), then certainly of the era into which he was born.

Psychology, psychiatry, and neurology, as we have seen, provide good examples of how science became the obsessive activity it did, and Freud can help us explore this issue. Unlike the physical sciences of zoology or comparative anatomy, in which one can trace a kind of clarification and increasingly accurate set of descriptions, the mental sciences have had less obvious success. Here the diagnoses change regularly; the cure rate remains fairly constant (and comparatively low compared to, say, the cure rate for testicular cancer); and the methods are always shifting without what might be called a quantifiable rate of success. Two approaches to the study of the mind have remained fairly consistent: that which seeks to find a structural, physical cause of mental illness (lesions, brain structure, brain chemistry, or electrical activity); and the dynamic explanations that rely on models of pressures, levels, conflicts, thoughts, feelings, perceptions, and misperceptions. The former is always material, and the latter is always psychological or metaphysical. Freud began with the former and quickly moved to the latter, as he tells us: "I passed from the histology of the nervous system, to neuropathology, and then, thanks to fresh influences, I began to be concerned with neuroses" (*SE* 20: 254).

We can say that Freud began with the anatomical sciences, and when he moved to the psychological and metaphysical, he tried to keep to a scientific base. As he wrote in 1895 in his early essay "Project for a Scientific Psychology," "The intention is to furnish a psychology that shall be a natural science, to represent psychical processes as quantitatively determinate states of specifiable material particles, thus making those processes perspicuous and free from contradiction" (*SE* 1:295). Freud's impulse was to combine the material and the dynamic by thinking of psychical processes (dynamic) as "material particles." This almost quantum theory of psychology aimed to give a "specifiable" materiality to the often elusory and chimerical theories of dynamic psychology. Freud seems to have believed that by showing that the mind followed scientific rules he could give a scientific patina to an area that might on some level be resistant to or transgressive of science, that might in fact reveal the inutility of science.

Yet the obsession of psychoanalysis wasn't purely located in the scientific method. The thinking was more or less magical. Freud's notion was that an idea, a single idea at that, could set you free. You didn't have to be a man or woman of science to be an analyst; because psychoanalysis was based on an insight, anyone could be an analyst, just as anyone could be a patient. When a colleague inquired who qualified to be an analyst, Freud responded, "Anyone who has recognized transference and resistance as the focal points of therapy belongs irretrievably to the mad horde" (*SE* 12:346). The fact that Freud saw, even in joking, that to be an analyst was in fact to be part of a "mad horde" is worth noting. Analyst and patient form a unit. You can't have psychoanalysis without that unit, and so, in some major sense, the analyst is as mad as the patient, and indeed perhaps mad because the aim of analysis was to return to one fixed point, to reveal that point, and have the patient see that point. In this sense, psychoanalysis is a glorified version of idée fixe.

NOTHING HAPPENS: THEY JUST TALK

Indeed, the breakthrough of psychoanalysis is that the continuing democratization of madness and the increasing consumerism linked to the rise of medicine can be nicely combined in one place. If we consider the quartet's institutionalization into the array of selected diseases from neurasthenia to hysteria, psychoanalysis domesticates the process of treatment and cure. Gone are the institutions, torture-like devices, moral regimens, and dietary restrictions, since, as Freud says, psychoanalysis does not require the patient to go to an institution or spa, but simply to see the doctor down the street or *strasse*. Thus psychoanalysis "leaves the patient in his environment and in his usual mode of life during the treatment." In fact, says Freud, "nothing takes place between them except that they talk to each other" (*SE* 20:187). In earlier regimens, there was much at stake—in the most extreme cases surgical operations and other dramatic interventions. To become a patient was to risk one's life and limb. But the invention of the psychoanalytic method was to make the process not only relatively harmless, but a kind of domestic occupation in which the patient is nestled into the comfort of a doctor's office, reclining on a couch or divan, and just speaking about whatever comes to mind. Thus, with Freud, consumerism meets convenience—one-stop therapeutic shopping.

The simple fact that nothing happens except that "they talk to each other" deepens the obsessive quality of both the disease and the cure. The talk is, paradoxically, not focused and ruminative but a kind of unfocused palaver for the initiated. Freud advises analysts to do the opposite of concentrate. Just as the patient is advised to say anything in analysis, the analyst is advised to take a mental state "of not focusing on anything in particular, but giving everything the same kind of 'impartially suspended attention,'" which is in essence to "rely completely on your 'unconscious memory.'" In other words, "you should listen and not worry whether you notice anything or not."[5] If the patient is talking without noticing and the analyst is listening without noticing, there is a strange kind of agreement proceeding.[6] It is as if, Freud mentions, the analyst's unconscious is attuned to that of the patient. This kind of attention recalls Matthew Arnold's notion of the critic as one who has a "disinterested love of a free play of the mind." Yet, instead of the result being a kind of unfocused ramble, Freud sees this activity as an essential part of the disinterested vision of science. "I cannot urge colleagues emphatically enough to take a leaf out of the surgeon's book during psychoanalytic treatment and, like him, put to one side all your emotions and even your human sympathies in order to concentrate your mental powers on a *single aim:* carrying out the operation as skillfully as possible"[7] (italics mine).

As to his own life, Freud stresses to his friend and correspondent Wilhelm Fliess that a man like him "cannot live without a hobby-horse, a consuming passion—in Schiller's words—a tyrant. . . . I have found one. In its service I know no limits. It is psychology."[8] Freud adds, "For me, however, nothing counts but my work, and I am prepared to become entirely single-minded if only I can carry it through."[9] Freud's own admission of his single aim or consuming passion seems confirmed in William James assessment of Freud: "I confess that he made on me personally the impression of a man obsessed with fixed ideas."[10]

Freud, in effect, creates a kind of thinking that is both paradoxical and yet characteristic of an age. The analyst must both focus in a single-minded way and at the same time refuse to focus. The paradox is that the open-mindedness is actually a form of activity geared to create single-mindedness. The single-mindedness applies both to the patient and to the analyst, who form a new bond as mental and emotional conjoined twins attached at the unconscious. The single-mindedness also applies to the ultimate goal of psychoanalysis, which is to uncover childhood repressions of the unconscious and of the drives. In this sense, the Freudian method continues in a line of nineteenth-century science as obsession—single-focus activities that study single-focus states of mind.

PSYCHOANALYSIS STARTS OUT WITH OBSESSION

Obsession, it turns out, is the originating portal into psychoanalysis. As one researcher notes, "Psychoanalytic understanding of obsessional neurosis on the one hand, and of hysteria on the other, can be seen as comprising the clinical keystones on which Freud constructed his understanding of the unconscious and its role in psychopathology."[11] It was through studying patients with obsessions that Freud arrived at the initial central insights of psychoanalysis. As he states in an early essay written in 1894, "After making a detailed study of a number of nervous patients suffering from phobias and obsessions, I was led to attempt an explanation of those symptoms; and this enabled me afterwards to arrive successfully at the origin of pathological ideas of this sort in new and different cases" (*SE* 3:45). Or as he put it in another essay, "I found that neurasthenia presented a monotonous clinical picture in which, as my analyses showed, a 'psychical mechanism' played no part. There was a sharp distinction between neurasthenia and 'obsessional neurosis,' the neurosis of obsessional ideas proper" (*SE* 2:258). It is noteworthy that in the former early essay, Freud uses the term "psychical analysis," but two years later he coined the term "psychoanalysis." We can then say that psychoanalysis literally came into being when Freud eschewed the monotonous recurrence of neurasthenia in favor of the "complicated psychical mechanism" (*SE* 2:258) of obsessional neurosis.[12]

ANXIETY ATTACKS EUROPE

Further, it was by separating what Freud called "anxiety neurosis" (*Angstneurose*) from neurasthenia that he left the physical symptoms behind and entered into the psychodynamic. Not uncoincidentally, his was the first use of the term "anxiety" in medicine, at least in English according to the *OED*. This connection between anxiety, obsession, phobias, and what, for want of a better term, we might call "modern consciousness" is significant. The problematics of obsession lead us in the direction of a society that is replete with people filled with obsessions and anxiety. This state, as Freud opined, was not confined to the sick or the degenerate but was more properly considered part of the range of the normal. Patients become obsessive and anxious in the context of a society that creates, notices, and even values—for diagnosis or cultural desiderata—those symptoms.

The emphasis on anxiety as a regnant symptom in the symptom pool is worth considering for a moment. It's important to realize that while we talk about anxiety or even worrying, we assume that people in the past have always had anxiety or worried, but both words actually arise in the modern sense in the nineteenth century. Adam Phillips has pointed out that the *OED* begins to cite "worrying" as a state of mind, as opposed to the thing that your cat does to its unfortunate mouse victim, in the nineteenth century. It is then that we see Dickens's characters "worriting," or worrying. As Phillips says, "Worry begins to catch on as a new state of mind."[13] We can see the rise of worrying and anxiety as part of the general stream of focus on nerves, nervousness, and their etiology from obsessive behaviors. Society, in effect, had to learn how to worry or how to organize a range of feeling into something it would call anxiety. Anxiety or angst then begins to show up in art, literature, and eventually film—think of the works of Poe, Kafka, Fritz Lang—where it can be a structuring device in genres like horror or suspense and can even become a commodity for which audiences will pay good money.

In an essay that appeared in French, Freud makes clear that he is talking about anxiety (*anxiété*) and not anguish (*angoisse*) (*SE* 3:75). The former notion of angst seems to be used as a more generic and abstract quality. Like obsession, anxiety fills the canvas of turn-of-the-century Europe captured best in Munch's *The Scream* or the work of Oskar Kokoschka, referred to as the "artist of angst" by Carl Schorske.[14] Freud's further contribution to the anxiety model was his use of the word "attack," as in "anxiety attack." The word "attack" began being used in English in the sense of a disease attacking by mid-nineteenth century. The *OED* also lists the first use of the word for military attacks a bit later in the century. Assuming Freud was aware of this new usage, he would have been linking the psychological and the physical in a new way—postulating that anxiety could be seen as both a disease and an aspect of modern warfare. In addition, Freud describes "a quantum of anxiety in a freely floating state" (*SE* 3:93). So anxiety moves from the world of affect to the world of medicine, becomes a universal state of being, joins the ills of disease, war, and the human condition, and is separated and isolated in some perhaps new way.[15]

One of the familiar ways that the nineteenth century understood anxiety was as the result of a shock. The literature of the period is filled with examples of shock leading to illness, fever, and mental distress. But Freud, counterintuitively, denies this aspect to anxiety neurosis and argues against his critic Leopold Löwenfeld's assertion that anxiety results from a specific frightening incident (*SE* 3:126ff). Freud instead traces anxiety back to his fixed point—sexual repression. By cutting off anxiety from general experience and allowing the concept of a free-floating anxiety that is purely the result of sexual repression, Freud clinched the obsessive nature of anxiety.

The reason I am stressing the importance of Freud's focus on anxiety is that this, at least initially, was the break that created the space for psychoanalysis. And this elevation of anxiety to the level of a cultural phe-

nomenon allowed Freud to generalize from neurasthenia, owned in effect
by Beard, to a new kind of neurosis that Freud himself controlled—and it
was through the idea of obsessional neurosis that he controlled it.

SEPARATING FROM CHARCOT: GROUNDWORK
FOR OBSESSIVE NEUROSIS

To understand Freud's trajectory from anatomy to the destiny of obsessional neurosis, we need to do a bit of biography. Freud began his medical
work as a young man working in the Institute of Comparative Anatomy.
He received in 1885, at the age of twenty-nine, a small sum of money to
go to Paris and study with the famous neurologist Jean-Martin Charcot.
He spent a year at Salpêtrière in what was the hotbed of the study of hysteria and nervous diseases. Young physicians from France and the rest
of Europe sat at Charcot's feet and learned his techniques. Charcot was
a very systematic man from whom Freud may have learned his method
of proceeding and analysis. Freud observed hysteria through Charcot's
well-known public demonstrations, which probably led him to the most
important work he did with Breuer. Yet Freud immediately parted from
Charcot, whom he admired greatly, in a telling footnote to a translation of
Charcot's Tuesday seminars. Freud added this footnote disagreeing with
a statement by Charcot that heredity was the "true cause" of a patient's
hysterical attacks, vertigo, and agoraphobia. Freud wrote, "I venture upon
a contradiction here. The more frequent cause of agoraphobia as well as
of most other phobias lies not in heredity but in abnormalities of sexual
life" (*SE* 1:139). Freud, in an early and deft move, switched the etiology of
hysteria from hereditary factors to sexual "abnormalities." Here we might
say is the obsessive move that inaugurated psychoanalysis proper.[16]

Freud presents to us "the psychological theory of obsessions and phobias" (*SE* 3:45) and in effect lays the groundwork for psychoanalysis. He
writes in an early paper,

> If someone with a disposition [to neurosis] lacks the aptitude for conver-
> sion, but if, nevertheless, in order to fend off an incompatible idea, he sets
> about separating it from its affect, then that affect is obliged to remain in
> the psychical sphere. The idea, now weakened, is still left in conscious-
> ness, separated from all association. But this affect, which has become
> free, attaches itself to other ideas which are not in themselves incompat-

ible; and thanks to this 'false connection,' those ideas turn into obsessional ideas. (3:51–52)

In other words, to use some later terminology, Freud arrives at the notion that by repressing the unwanted idea, defined as "really distressing experiences in the subject's sexual life which he is striving to forget" (3:75), and splitting it from its associated affect, that affect will attach itself to other ideas which will, by the force of that affect, become obsessional.

The system so developed is actually a kind of mini-obsession in itself, with a hyperawareness of thought processes and the willingness to break them down to very small component parts. There is too a conservation of energy that postulates that nothing is lost, or can be lost, and all is therefore recoverable. In psychoanalytic theory, in other words, there is no forgetting or absent-mindedness. If you forget, your psyche will remember. If your psyche forgets, the analyst will remember. This singleness of vision, this faith in the recurrence of ideas or affects, is what is characteristic of Freud's conceptualization at this point.

One of the driving forces tied to the problematics of obsession was the concept of degeneration. A seesaw of opinion rose and fell concerning the partially insane—were they insane because they were degenerate or were they degenerate because they were insane? Since, as we saw, Freud rejected the hereditarian impulse of Charcot, he was led to redefine insanity into neurosis in the broadest sense, in order that it ultimately include every civilized person. Obsession allowed Freud to expand the numbers of those who might be obsessive, saying that they were "no more degenerate than the majority of neurotics . . . because they sometimes improve, and sometimes, indeed, we even succeed in curing them" (SE 3:74). Thus, because obsessives were not incurables and were not degenerates, they were in effect somewhat "normal."

But the somewhat "normal" has to be totally redefined in a Freudian model. Eugenics and moral physiology had been developing a way of talking about sexual hygiene that promoted a new vision of a normal sexual life. Indeed, there was a struggle over the concept of the normal, particularly as regards human sexuality. Freud achieves this redefinition of normality through an obsessive rumination on the very concept. In his refutation of Löwenfeld, Freud notes that his insistence on a sexual etiology for anxiety neurosis is not disproved by Löwenfeld's example of a woman who seemed normal and developed anxiety over a fright. Freud responds by questioning whether the woman did indeed have a normal *vita sexualis:* "Which of all these elements were present in Löwenfeld's case? I do not know. But I repeat: this case is evidence against me only if the lady who responded to a single fright with an anxiety neurosis had before then enjoyed a normal *vita sexualis*" (*SE* 3:129). The catch of course is that under Freud's scrutiny, there is no one who has a normal sexual life, and so, in yet another way, neurosis becomes endemic. Thus through obsessive observation of and rumination on the (by definition always) hidden sexual life of the bourgeoisie in Vienna and elsewhere, obsession deriving from anxiety deriving from sexuality will always surface.

FREUD AS COMPULSIVE WRITER

Like Zola, Freud was a prolific writer. His life was an obsession of work and writing that amounted to a distinct monomania. Lydia Flem observes in her biography, "Freud lived pen in hand; he writes everywhere, all the time, and has always done so."[17] Freud's entire day was spent working. He saw patients in the morning and afternoon, and he wrote at night—usually until two or three in the morning. Freud saw himself as a writer, and admitted to a visitor, "Ever since childhood, my secret hero has been Goethe. . . . I have been able to win my destiny in an indirect way and have attained my dream: to remain a man of letters, though still in appearance a doctor."[18] To be a man of letters is, at this point, to engage in a variety of graphomania in which work, thought, and writing all come together. As Freud noted, "I really can't imagine that a life without work would be comfortable to me: fantasizing and work are one and the same for me and nothing else is fun for me." But, as happened to the characters in *L'oeuvre,* work can haunt one. As Freud continues, "That would be a recipe for happiness if it were not for the horrible thought that productivity is entirely dependent on one's being in the right mood. What can one begin on a day, or during a period of time, in which thoughts fail one or words don't come? It is impossible to stop trembling at this possibility."[19] Freud amplifies this point, saying, "I should have been sure of myself throughout my life if I could have been sure of productive capacity at all times and in all moods. Unfortunately, this has never been the case. There have always been days in between when nothing could come and when I have been in danger of losing all ability to work and to struggle, owing to certain minor fluctuations in mood and physical health."[20] Like Zola, although Freud writes obsessively, he sees himself as unproductive and lives in dread of those times when he cannot write. Indeed, his addictive use of cocaine was largely the result of his trying to dispel moods of severe depression that kept him from writing.[21] Freud's recourse to cocaine, which essentially jumpstarted his career in midlife, was to ensure the productivity of his writing and thinking.

Many critics, including Steven Marcus, have noted that the case history is not an independent form but relies heavily on other kinds of narratives—most notably the ascendant form of the nineteenth century, the novel. Freud's desire to write and Zola's desire to be a scientist link both thinkers into this narrative mode of analysis. In fact, Freud mentions to a friend, "In my mind, I always construct novels, using my experience as a psychoanalyst; my wish is to become a novelist."[22]

CAUGHT IN THE RAT MAN'S OBSESSIVE TRAP

Freud's writing compulsion and ruminative, obsessive thinking come together in his essay on the "Rat Man," which was fully titled "Notes upon a Case of Obsessional Neurosis," published early in his career in 1909. Indeed, the opening of the case of the Rat Man sounds like the beginning of a nineteenth-century novel with the narrator's setting of the scene: "A youngish man of university education introduced himself to me with the statement that he had suffered from obsessions ever since his childhood" (SE 10:158). Like many narrators, Freud does not tell us anything about himself directly, thereby adding an element of omniscience and control.

Freud plunges in the first paragraph into the erotic biography of this young man, who reports that his "sexual life had been stunted;[23] onanism had played only a small part in it, in his sixteenth or seventeenth year. His potency was normal: he had first had intercourse at the age of twenty-six" (SE 10:158). The Rat Man himself presents immediately his own sexual biography. When Freud asks him why he had chosen to present this information in the beginning of the conversation, the Rat Man replies that he is familiar with Freud's theories, although he also admits that he has never read any of Freud's work. What we see is a good example of how the symptom pool works—patients present their symptoms through a process of interacting with cultural expectations and discursive knowledge in society. Freud's desire to include this fact also now indicates that awareness of his own ideas is infiltrating a certain segment of society, in effect changing the symptom pool. Thus, obsession is not only a symptom of the Rat Man but also a symptom of Freudianism.

Freud begins the therapy by explaining the condition of the treatment—the Rat Man is advised "to say everything that came into his head" (*SE* 10:159). But it is not only the Rat Man who must do so, but Freud as well. Indeed, there is a kind of literary narrative style that we've seen with Zola—the faith that just sitting down and writing will produce something worthwhile. Recall that Zola, after preparation, wrote steadily and without revision. He never reread his works. In Freud's case, his advice to "say everything" was also part of his writing technique. Some have speculated that Freud's advice to "say everything" came from a book he had read in his youth, *The Art of Becoming an Original Writer in Three Days,* by Ludwig Börne. When Freud was thirteen he received this book, which later he recalled "could really be the source of my originality."[24] According to Freud, Borne advised that one could become a good writer if one took "a few sheets of paper and for three days on end write down without fabrication or hypocrisy, everything that comes into your head . . . and when three days have passed you will be quite out of your senses with astonishment at the new and unheard-of thoughts you have had." As Flem notes, "Freud neglects to mention this advice applies not only to his patients . . . but to his own work of putting thoughts into words" (98). Freud wrote rather quickly, often several papers at once, and the nature of his writing, while organized to a degree, is often quite rambling and associative (103).

In this early case history of the Rat Man, this own associative method of writing has to be tempered by a reality—the story is ultimately the clinical history of the Rat Man. As he says, "What follows is based upon notes made on the evening of the day of treatment and adheres as closely as possible to my recollection of the patient's words" (*SE* 10:159). The issue here is how to record after the fact the patient's words to get as close as possible to what the patient actually said. Freud chose this after-the-fact method because it was the least distracting to the patient, since distraction can do the patient "more harm than can be made up for by any increase in accuracy" (*SE* 10:159). We begin to see here a specific obsessive worry developing in Freud that goes alongside his compulsive command to "say everything"—how to record faithfully what the patient said, to repeat everything that came into the patient's head, while also being attentive to the patient at the moment of utterance? If one distracts the patient by recording what is going on at the moment, one loses the connection between the patient's and the analyst's unconscious. But if one doesn't, one loses the contact with the immediate and accurate words of the patient, which are the outward manifestations of the structure of the unconscious. This paradox amounts to a Freudian version of the Heisenberg uncertainty principle—you can't have accurate recording and accurate analysis at the same time.

Freud's solution to record after the fact sacrifices accuracy for analysis. In that sense, the method is more likely to allow Freud himself, rather than the patient, to be the final one to "say everything." In essence, we are not getting the Rat Man verbatim so much as Freud's version of what he remembers about the Rat Man. At the same time, here is the beginning of a pattern of worrying, of obsessing, on Freud's part that is partly a reflection of his own obsession with "saying all" and also a reflection of the Rat Man's obsessive thinking. In Freudian terms, Freud's countertransference produces a duplication of the symptomatology of the patient in the therapist.

This obsession takes a somewhat devious form that has to do with how Freud should tell the story as narrative. Freud the writer bumps up against Freud the analyst. In the case of the former, the aim is to record what was said; in the latter to interpret it helpfully for the patient. But the contradiction is that for Freud successfully to be the writer (with his own associative method) he has to work over the patient's narrative. Whose associations will dominate; whose version will become the official narrative? One sees in this attempt to write all the words down, to get them right, a continuation of the attention to writing and words that produced, among other things, the graphomania of the more than twenty thousand letters Freud produced, many of which are to a recipient who is also the object of obsessive love or attention, notably first Fliess, who was then displaced by Jung.

In the Rat Man story, we are presented with seeming random reminiscences of the patient. He has obsessive thoughts, that is to say, thoughts he cannot stop thinking about. This includes at age four or five "a burning and tormenting curiosity to see the female body," at six the "morbid idea that my parents knew my thoughts," and the notion that "something must happen if I thought such things" (*SE* 10: 160–62). Freud sees these thoughts as part of a "complete obsession neurosis, wanting no essential element" (*SE* 10:162). For Freud, this early complete nucleus of neurosis fits in with his ideas of the erotic life of children and its effect on later neurosis. "Obsessional neuroses make it much more obvious than hysterias that the factors which go to form a psychoneurosis are to be found in the patient's infantile sexual life and not in his present one" (*SE* 10:165).

Here again is the key insight that allows Freud to carve out the difference between psychoanalysis and other psychiatric endeavors: first, the problem begins, fully formed, in childhood sexual life; second, the route to neuroses isn't hysteria—it's obsession.

We might point here to the underlying reflexive obsession of Freud, that when an explanation for behavior is sought, the answer will always lie in the sexual. There is required a focused gaze that will find the underlying erotic disturbance: "the current sexual life of an obsessional neurotic may often appear perfectly normal to a superficial observer"(*SE* 10:165). However, the trained eye will see the abnormality. One of Freud's favorite writers was Arthur Conan Doyle, and with good reason, since Sherlock Holmes's investigative gaze would always pick out the seemingly superficial and irrelevant clues or details to arrive at the underlying, hidden narrative of murder or theft. Both Holmes and Freud will need to be hypervigilant in trying to locate and interpret seemingly irrelevant or obvious clues.

Two more apparently insignificant stories ensue in the Rat Man's analysis—both initiated by a captain during maneuvers. One is about rats used in torture in the "East," and this story is perhaps the most related to the Rat Man's eponymous fear of rats. A second story involves the patient having ordered a set of pince-nez by mail. The same captain who told him about the rat torture also mentioned that the pince-nez had arrived at the post office and that a Lieutenant A had paid the shipping charges and therefore should be repaid. The patient goes on to provide a detailed story about the captain's suggestion that he repay Lieutenant A the very small sum of money involved. The Rat Man then had the obsessive thought that he should not pay the lieutenant. A long and tortuous story follows in which the patient both tries to and tries not to repay the debt.

Freud goes to great lengths to get the story right, even though, he notes, "it would not surprise me to hear that at this point the reader had ceased to be able to follow" (*SE* 10:169). The fact is that almost no reader can actually follow the details of the story, and as a novelist Freud might well have left out the details. Whenever I have asked my students to try to recreate a coherent narrative from the Rat Man's story, they are unable to do so. But acting as a psychoanalyst, of course, Freud cannot leave any detail out, given the obsessive nature of the observations and conclusions required. So Freud attempts to engage in "straightening out the various distortions involved in his story" (*SE* 10:172). He discovers various facts and people who had been left out of the patient's narrative, but on adding these corrective details, Freud notes, "I must admit that when this correction has been made this behaviour becomes even more senseless and unintelligible than before" (*SE* 10:173). Ironically, Freud himself now is caught in this narrative web, not only by being forced to decipher something that is undecipherable, but also by becoming a minor character in the story itself, since the patient came to Freud's office ostensibly to get a certificate from a medical doctor that would force Lieutenant A to accept the money as a medical necessity. The Rat Man's obsession to pay the lieutenant back now sucks the analyst Freud into the ruminative whirlwind.

As a narrator, Freud faces a problem. He's already confused his reader by obsessively pouring over the overwhelming detail that the Rat Man provided in his session. The neat narrative thing to do now would be to "solve" the problem and make things intelligible, but Freud tells us, "The reader must not expect to hear at once what light I have to throw upon the patient's strange and senseless obsessions about the rats." The reason he can't solve the problem is that "the true technique of psychoanalysis requires the physician to suppress his curiosity and leave the patient complete freedom in choosing the order in which topics shall succeed each other during the treatment" (*SE* 10:173–74). Of course, this a narrative ruse, in a sense, since nothing prevents Freud from taking the path of least resistance and putting the Rat Man's narrative in proper order for the readers. But his obsession with the dynamics of recording the detail and telling the story, which at this early date in the history of psychoanalysis is really an attention to the technique of psychoanalysis itself, forces Freud (and us) to go further into the obsessive maze of the Rat Man's ruminative thinking.

After more recalled incidents, Freud begins to provide an "explanation" for the obsessional ideas. We should recall that Freud wrote this essay in 1909, and so we can see this work as part of a more general project of explaining unlikely and ineffable phenomena like dreams, symptoms, jokes, slips of the tongue—all seemingly irrelevant and without the possibility of explanation. We have to recall that although we are now used to such "Freudian" explanations, in his own time the idea of explaining ephemeral epiphenomena such as these would have be strange and unlikely. So, Freud writes, "obsessional ideas, as is well known, have an appearance of being either without motive or without meaning, just as dreams do" (*SE* 10:186). But given Freud's belief (we might say delusion) that all things have meaning, he notes that "the problem of translating them [obsessional ideas] may seem insoluble; but we must never let ourselves be misled by that illusion. The wildest and most eccentric obsessional or compulsive ideas can be cleared up if they are investigated deeply enough" (*SE* 10:186). The matter of depth is what is significant—a deep investigation, a very deep investigation, will produce a result. Of course, this is a tautological explanation, since the only adequate result will be that which is produced by a deep enough investigation to yield the sexual substrate.

THE RAT MAN'S OBSESSION FOR UNDERSTANDING

In this case, Freud's manner of proceeding is to place things in temporal order—so that the obsession is brought into contact with the circumstances surrounding it when it first came to light. Freud describes some various obsessions of the Rat Man, but one in particular stands out—an "obsession for understanding." This annoying behavior was part of an attempt to "understand the precise meaning of every syllable that was addressed to him, as though he might otherwise be missing some priceless treasure. Accordingly he kept asking: 'What was it you said just then?' and after it had been repeated to him he could not help thinking it sounded different the first time" (*SE* 10:190). It doesn't take much perspicacity to see some kind of mirror in this to Freud's own method in which the desire to understand at all costs, the need for repetition, the hyperawareness of words and their meanings is paramount. This mania recalls Esquirol's definition of "reasoning monomania."[25] Albert Hirst, a patient of Freud, noted that Freud "would be very active and inquisitive about loose ends, invariably asking for explanations of whatever he did not understand or whatever was incompletely presented. Once, when Hirst attempted to withhold details of a sexual incident involving a member of his family, Freud demanded a complete account."[26] This behavior recalls the Rat Man's compulsion to understand. As Freud notes in his Wolf Man article, "It is always a strict law of dream interpretation that an explanation must be found for every detail." (*SE* 17:42n1).

The Rat Man, in effect, becomes a kind of exaggerated version of Freud himself, no doubt one of the reasons that Freud is drawn to explain this case history so extensively. In doing so, Freud extends Hamlet's observation "Nothing is, but thinking makes it so." For Freud, doubting, wondering, trying to understand, brooding becomes an erotic activity. "The thought-process itself becomes sexualized, for the sexual pleasure which is normally attached to the content of thought becomes shifted on to the act of thinking itself, and the gratification derived from reaching the conclusion of a line of thought is experienced as a sexual gratification" (*SE* 10:245). This definition of the pleasure of overthinking, thinking too much, resonates with Freud's overthinking of this case. In recounting the Rat Man's obsessive tale, Freud tells the story of the pince-nez no less than three times, repeating the details, including the seemingly irrelevant detail of the 3.80 florins in question. Freud is so involved in the telling and retelling, that he involves not only the reader, but also his editors, the Stracheys. Freud notes that "my account of it [the Rat Man's story] may have failed to clear it up entirely." To make things clearer the editors encouraged Freud to place a map showing the location of the various events in the story. Freud notes, "My translators have justly observed that the patient's behaviour remains unintelligible" without further details. But the map and the details do little to make things clearer.[27]

The problem is that a massive countertransference has occurred in which Freud's own obsessiveness, an obsessiveness that laid the foundations for psychoanalysis, has become exacerbated in his treatment of the Rat Man. Freud vacillates from being unable to explain or even record, to providing the "solution" and "explanation" of what is hidden.[28] At one point he notes, "I must confess that I can only give a very incomplete account of the whole business [of the symbolic meaning of rats]" (*SE* 10:213). At another he recognizes that his own and the patient's associations are somewhat far-fetched: "If the reader feels tempted to shake his head at the possibility of such leaps of imagination in the neurotic mind, I may remind him that artists have sometimes indulged in similar freaks of fancy" (*SE* 10:214n1). It is unclear at this point whether Freud is saying that the Rat Man or he himself is the artist. The essay ends by noting that "my communication is incomplete in every sense" (*SE* 10:248). I am not the first to comment on Freud's taking on the obsessive behavior exhibited by the Rat Man,[29] but the point I want to make is that Freud's getting lost in the details is a consequence of his two contradictory aims—the obsession to say everything and the obsession to explain everything. There is the further contradiction of Freud's desire to record the exact details of his patient saying everything. And that obsession spills over to the editors of the Standard Edition, who found and included Freud's original case notes for the Rat Man's analysis, as well as the legions of scholars, this one included, who then have tried obsessively to make sense or coherence from this intellectual hologram of obsessionality.

BEGINNING AND ENDING WITH OBSESSION

In his obsession to trace obsession, Freud returned to the subject at the end of his career, and wrote that "obsessional neurosis is unquestionably the most interesting and repaying subject of analytic research" (*SE* 20:113). Still haunted by it in 1926, as he was in one of his earliest papers, "The Neuro-Psychoses of Defence," written in 1893, Freud remains in an obsessive-compulsive repetition, noting that "as a problem it has not yet been mastered" (*SE* 20:113), and that "obsessional neurosis presents such a vast multiplicity of phenomena that no efforts have yet succeeded in making a coherent synthesis of all its variations" (*SE* 20:118). One can only ask, "How could anyone make a coherent system out of system that is obsessed with coherence?" The devil would always be in the details.

In the end, we see how significant it is that Freud's career is bookended, as it were, by speculations about OCD. Why is that? One reason might be found in the connection between obsessive neurosis and "analysis." Freud used the term "analysis" for the first time in the "Neuro-Psychoses" essay. The *OED* informs us that the word had been used for quite a long time before that to mean "the resolution or breaking up of anything complex into its various simple elements." The term had been used since the sixteenth century in the realms of chemistry, optics, literature, grammar, mathematics, and logic. But the new usage, which pops up in the 1880s and 1890s, is related to philosophy and psychology. In the latter case, the word means "the mental process of discrimination, by separate attention, of the separable elements in a totality of simultaneous sensory impressions, or in any other complex experience" (*OED*, s.v.). One of the first to use the term was William James in 1890, three years before Freud used it. We can assume that Freud saw himself as using an au courant term that had resonance with philosophy and psychology rather than psychiatry, neurology, or medicine. We might also want to recall that literary analysis, in its more modern sense of "critical analysis of text" starts being used in German and English around the 1860s. Given Freud's proclivity to see himself as a man of letters, a crypto-novelist, a philosopher, this use of "analysis" makes sense.

Further, analysis implies a rigorous method that involves close, single-minded attention. When Freud begins to analyze the Rat Man's text, he engages in this obsessive activity that is increasingly becoming a hallmark of the modern. We can think of psychoanalysis as a legitimate form of obsessive neurosis—a sublimation or an intellectualization or rationalization of the very thing it is studying.[30]

In the idea of analysis, we have a nodal point that connects our discussion of Zola and Freud. The scientific study of Zola—that is the study of Zola by scientists and the study by Zola of inherited traits in his novel's characters—merges with Freud's analysis of the Rat Man and his own project of psychoanalysis. Further, Zola saw his own novelistic task as a form of analysis. In a more general sense, one could speculate that one characteristic of the modern world was the incorporation of science into a system previously dominated by the humanities and theology. That is, the intrusion or adaptation of analysis into a belleletristic world signaled a change in the way knowledge was organized and perceived.

Indeed, in the United States, the growth and change of the university was linked to this incorporation of science. Daniel Coit Gilman, who reformed higher education in the United States in the mid-nineteenth century, made his first dramatic change by creating a school of science within Yale, the University of California, and Johns Hopkins.[31] Coinciding with the emphasis on science was the reformation of the study of the humanities, so that scholars thought more like scientists and less like theologians. George Santayana, who taught philosophy at Harvard from 1889 until 1912, wrote that "many of the younger professors of philosophy are no longer the sort of persons that might as well have been clergymen or schoolmasters: they have rather the type of mind of a doctor."[32] Freud and Zola are both men of this type—writers who are scientists; scientists who are writers. Both engage in analysis of language and texts looking for scientific solutions. The modality of the way they know and what they want to know about is, in short, obsessive.

6

Obsessive Sex and Love

When I talk to people about the book I am writing on obsession, they usually give me a nod and a wink. They assume, like Freud, that obsession is actually, when all is said and done, about sex. Obsession and sex seem to go together like a horse and carriage, or like a stalker and a victim. While sex seems the case in point for obsession, obsession is a much more global concept, as I have tried to show, than is obsessive sex. Yet this book would be missing what is in effect the "money shot" if it didn't bring obsessive sexuality into the picture. If, as we've seen, obsession is the motor of disciplinarity, the object of disciplinary study, and increasingly a cultural abnormal state that everyone seeks as a norm—then we can understand how doing too much of one thing came to apply to sexuality and love as well as to work or thinking.

THE CULTURAL GOAL

So what is obsessive love? How can we count the ways? We could divide it up, like a truly obsessive observer, into categories. First, there is a generally held cultural notion of passion beyond passion, the trembling, ecstatic, dangerous, hypnotic kind of sex that is a feature of novels, movies, and fantasies whispered in the dark. We might define this kind of sex as a matter of an intensified degree and think of it in relation to something we might culturally regard as "normal" sex. That latter category, as we will see, is an intensely fraught one. But in opposition to mad, obsessive passion, it represents the baseline for sex. Normal sex is more of obsessive sex's opposite than is, for example, chastity or anesthesia or anhedonia. Mad, passionate, obsessive sex is, in addition, the antidote or the polar opposite of humdrum sex, quotidian, uninspired, often conjugal, sex.

But how do we know about this dichotomy? If nothing else, our culture has done an excellent job of displaying the alternative between one and the other, casting both as knowable and certain states. We may have experienced the heights of one and the nadir of the other ourselves. No form of individual behavior is ever really outside biocultural influence. Even in the intensely personal realm of sexuality, we are constantly interpreting our bodily states, physical information, in larger cultural terms.

Perhaps the ads for Calvin Klein's perfume Obsession most directly capture the mood invoked by contemporary notions of obsession in love. Dimly lit pictures in monochromatic colors reveal aspects of bodies, often in combinations considered transgressive (that would be any more than two). Nudity, darkness, moisture, almost anything other than the missionary position, signal a sexuality beyond the bounds of the norm. Two men and a woman, a group of nude people wandering a surreal landscape, a man crouching next to a female torso his lips on her navel (fig. 6), a nude man and woman standing up on a swing, genitals pressed against each other.

The Calvin Klein ads, and many others for perfumes with names like Nude, Opium, Chaleur, tell us that obsession in the realm of sexuality is no vice. Indeed, in common parlance, for sexuality to be potent and satisfying it should verge on obsession, if not entirely depend on it. A popular book on obsession directed toward female readers states:

> I should make it clear that I am talking about one particular kind of love: romantic, obsessive love, the hot thing we fall into, the love we're all expected to experience and that we call true love. Think of novels like *Wuthering Heights* and *Dr. Zhivago,* or films like *Casablanca* and *The English Patient.* . . . What they have in common is this: two people obsessed with each other while all the ordinariness of life, its consolations and diversions, vanishes.[1]

The writer adds that "the story of obsessive love is a story about wanting something so badly that we will risk everything to gain it. As we hurtle

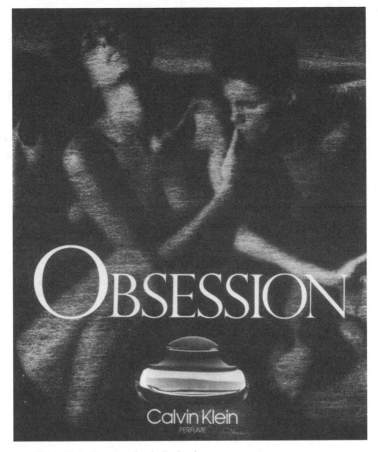

FIGURE 6. Calvin Klein Obsession for the Body ad.

down the highway at break-neck speed to meet our lover, as we defy all pre-scriptions for rational behavior, we are living a drama, and nothing else in the world matters. The puzzle is how we attach such life-and-death inten-sity to our feelings for these persons, since, after the obsession has played itself out, often these same persons stand before us almost as strangers."[2] This kind of pulse-racing, mind-fogging sexuality is the heroin-charged version of the quotidian aspirin most of us take as our sexual dose.

Advertising claims to promote this dark, secret kind of sexual involve-ment, but this is a high-fashion sexuality with models who are attractive to each other (presumably) and to as many other potential consumers as possible. The settings are either abstract or minimalist architecturally, usually linking sex to wealth and power. The models don't have to speak and reveal what they think or feel or their regional accents—they are timeless representatives of a privileged, mostly white, culture, or if darker, then they are required to have a metrosexual, cosmopolitan look. Yet, while they have taut and athletic bodies, they do not have genitals—and in that sense speak more of a polymorphous, over-the-top sexuality than they do of a reproductive or heteronormative kind.

This type of advertising favored by Calvin Klein is one that shifts the notion of obsession from attraction to a single person to attraction to a single hazy object—sexuality. One has no sense, in the ads, that any particular model has any specific interest in any other. Indeed, fashion models are notable for their interchangeability, even when they have their own personal signature. The models are presumably enthralled by the bodies of the other models, by the atmosphere of the sensual, and by some self-defining notion of being transgressive and excessive sexually. They are cool, detached actants caught in the repetition of an endless, preorgasmic loop.

NORMAL VS. OBSESSIVE SEX—INTENSITY, FREQUENCY, TYPE

As part of the development of sexuality as obsession, society has to form a distinction between legal and illegal sexual activities, which in turn helps to define and create sexual norms. You can't have obsession if you don't have a clear sense of normality. Obsessive behavior exists in dynamic tension with normal behavior, each shaping and defining the other. As with other forms of obsession, sexuality is divided into the culturally desirable goal to be attained and the quasi-criminal or actually criminal behavior to be avoided. In this split, mad passion is the hypostatized ideal, and stalking, sexual homicide, sexual addiction are the denigrated versions of this behavior. Dante gets kudos and John Hinckley Jr. gets life in prison.

Part of the mythology of obsessive love is grounded in a variety of cultural wish fulfillments. The wish is the collective antidote to the more practical knowledge that obsessive love is impossible to sustain, that that kind of intensity and frequency is more properly recognized as a moment in a relationship to be replaced by duty, responsibility, and some kind of purified but low-wattage radiance that carries people into the golden years. But moments can refuse to die, as the cultural wish implies. Such moments keep a phantasmatic and fantastical ghostly image that can lead to a determined attempt to recreate and sustain what culture asserts is both sustainable and yet unsustainable. Advertisements in the literary sections of respectable newspapers promise the rebirth of passionate sexuality through the diligent application of techniques learned by DVD. You're never too old or inexperienced to have obsessive sex.

Besides obsession in degree or intensity, there is obsession in relation to frequency—numbers of partners, numbers of orgasms within a number of hours or days, frequency of masturbation, and so on. Both degree and frequency are proscribed in the constructed version of normal sexuality because intensifying them can lead to a kind of sexuality that is hyper-focused, that takes up hours or days of psychic and physical time. "Doing one thing too much," the hallmark of nineteenth-century fears about obsession, is the cautionary watchword guarding against excessive sexuality. As an early sexologist writes in 1926, "The fundamental principle of hygiene . . . decrees that it is *never* good to make any *one* function of any organism, even the most important function, so predominant and absorbing that the others—the whole entity—suffer thereby. . . . This means that the highest development of mutual relationship on the sexual side must not invade and impair their mental life in common, and their psychic sympathy and partnership."[3] Obsessive passion in this sense can unhinge a couple, as it does, in novels like Zola's *Thérèse Raquin,* films like *Body Heat* or *Fatal Attraction,* or even contemporary cautionary tales like Michael Ryan's memoir *Secret Life* or Caveh Zahedi's film *I Am a Sex Addict,* where passion leads to irresponsibility, addiction, even murder and madness.

In addition to the categories of intensity and frequency is the grouping of kind or type. This group delimits the object of desire—who or what one loves: a woman, a man, both, a child, a horse, a shoe. Here we see the long-lived obsession with perversion—the origin of the word comes from a notion of "misdirection." Thus according to early sexologists the natural path of sexuality is always toward reproduction, and any diversion is literally a perversion of the reproductive function. The sperm cell is perverted in its goal of the ovum. Their reasoning was logical because of their evolutionary assumption that the sexual instinct is primarily a powerful one because it is yoked to the perpetuation of the species. The path of human male semen flows inevitably toward the womb of a human female, and when that stream is diverted or perverted, its goal is obscured. Inversion, perversion, homosexuality, as well as erotomania, autoeroticism, nymphomania, and so on fall into this category. If one loves the object too much, especially if the object is oneself or one's own genitalia, then this is an aspect of "kind." The preservation of semen and of its reproductive goal is not a prescriptive one in the nineteenth century, but actually descriptive, given the understanding of the function of sexuality as the royal road to reproduction.

EROTOMANIA

One longstanding and historically well-known "kind" of obsessive love has to do with a beloved who is unattainable and/or rejecting. Known as unrequited love or erotomania ("raving love"), it is described by the ancients, including Plautus, Plutarch, Galen, Paul Aegineta, Valerius Maximus, Amatus Lusitanus, Valleriola, Sennert, Tulpius, and others. Love sickness of this sort was linked to physical ailments and psychic distress. Arabic medicine brought the notion of unrequited love leading to general disease to medieval Europe and remained in European thought through the middle of the eighteenth century.[4] Called *amor heroes* in the twelfth century by physicians, and "erotic melancholy" by later ones, by the Renaissance it was seen as "a somatic disease of inflamed and congested genitals leading to disordered fantasy."[5] The most dramatic aspect of lovesickness is a devotion and obsession with the object of affection. Indeed it is possible to think of all obsession as a type and pattern of lovesickness. As André Du Laurens wrote in the sixteenth century, "The sillie loving worme cannot any more look upon any thing but his idol: al the functions of the bodie are likewise perverted, he becommeth pale, lean, souning."[6] This single-minded devotion to a love object to an excessive degree is the thing that launches obsessive love. But obsessive love will end up in our time not with a single person but a single purpose—addiction to sexuality.

A telling moment in this journey is Rousseau's *Confessions,* when, for the first time, a memoir confides in its readers the nature of a sexual obsession. Rousseau knows enough to signal to his readers that his behavior and revelation are memorable, worthy of writing about, and notable, as they have been, from his time to ours. Rousseau's confession is the guilty telling through a writerly bravado of how a moment in time became fixed as a moment in sensibility. Rousseau recounts an early experience of being spanked as a child that led to a lifelong preoccupation. He could not have an orgasm with a woman unless he was spanked. It's hard to imagine that previous writers could define themselves so strongly in terms of a particular sexual obsession. Rousseau along with De Sade move us from lovesickness, as the infatuation with a single beloved, to a process—sexuality as pain.

By the mid-eighteenth century the central focus of medicine on love and sexuality shifted from the symptoms of unrequited love, the wrong or failed object, to the dangers of excessive sexual appetite. We now move from kind to degree, as physicians become concerned about doing one thing too much in the sexual sphere. By the nineteenth century, erotomania changes its sense from unrequited love to nymphomania and satyriasis. The growing materialist bent of psychiatry came to see these behaviors as "diseases" located specifically in the genitals. Probably the first to describe this was William Cullen, who distinguished such sexual obsessions from his more general definition of neuroses, or general diseases of the nervous system. Nymphomaniacs and/or men with satyriasis were so not because of their minds or nerves, but because their genitals were abnormal. Cullen's diagnosis was perhaps based on M.-D.-T. de Bienville's definition of "uterine furor" as "a disorganized movement of the fibres in the female organs."[7] This localized explanation would remain through the twentieth century, when, for example, women who were highly sexed or lesbians were seen as such because of the size of their clitorises.[8]

DESIRE AS DISEASE

If nymphomania was a disease of frequency, masturbation became a disease of frequency, kind, and degree.[9] The history of the medicalization of masturbation provides us with a kind of master class on how medicine organized sexual behavior into the various types of obsession. The fear was that the masturbator had chosen the wrong object, was performing the behavior too much, and was too focused on the activity and the organ. In this sense, masturbation, as well as homosexuality and lesbianism, added another concept to degree and frequency, and that was object or kind. Desiring to have sex with oneself, with someone of the same gender, with any body part other than the penis or vagina, or with pain rather than pleasure presented an obsession of kind. Too much, too intensely, now joined with perverted aim. Thus masturbators, homosexuals, and nymphomaniacs/satyriasists were perverts, inverts, and so on, enjoying a practice that misdirected the obvious aim of sexuality, which was repro-duction. Where earlier some of these practices were seen as morally rep-rehensible or sacrilegious, they now became part of a new disease entity— diseases of sexuality.

Indeed, we might be able to say that sexuality became a disease. Fol-lowing the pattern that Georges Canguilhem described, medical science focused on the hypo/hyper dichotomy, best illustrated in blood sugar lev-els, and applied this model to sexuality.[10] This model defines illness by a matter of degree. If you have too much or too little blood sugar, you have an illness. Where you draw the line for normality is somewhat arbitrary. This was essentially the model of nineteenth-century views on sexuality, which constructed a norm of sexual behavior based in part on observation and on culturally embedded and often gendered, homophobic, ableist, and racialized notions of the body. Once this normal range was created, it was relatively easy to slide the gauge along the continuum to define too frequent, too intense, too aberrant.

Obsession as a matter of degree, frequency, or kind is thus turned into a physical disease, treated by doctors, particularly by gynecologists, who now consolidated their professional status through the management of such diseases. It became their role to create a complexly organized gradi-ent running from normal to abnormal sexuality. Consequently the nine-teenth century saw the rise of sexology and sexuality as discursive enti-ties.[11] Foucault and others see sexuality as invented, in this sense, in the nineteenth century insofar as "what we have come to call 'sexuality' is the product of a system of psychiatric knowledge."[12] Obviously, this is not to say that people didn't have sex before that time or didn't know they were having sex, but sexuality became a studied, human phenomenon set off from categories like "lust" or the physiology of the body. The word "sexu-ality" was first used in English in 1879 in reference to humans. Along with the appearance of this medicalized sexuality came the scientific study of norms and aberrations, most notably in the catalog of sexual perversions developed by Krafft-Ebing, Havelock Ellis, and other nineteenth- and early twentieth-century practitioners. Indeed, the work of sexology in this period was in fact an obsessive cataloging of sexual "perversions," often compiled to aid in criminal and judicial matters. It is exhausting to read works like Krafft-Ebing's *Psychopathia Sexualis*, filled with page after page of cataloged and subheaded sexual practices. The study of the obsessive in sexuality, as in other realms, requires the mirror image of the fixated observer who exhaustively catalogs the range of diseases that he in fact invents by creating such categories.

EXPERTS FOCUS ON SEX

It's not just that sex became a medicalized problem; it became a social problem as well. The focus was on obsessive sexuality, but it also was on an obsessive attention to sexuality by a new breed of experts. While many of those experts were scientists, there was a popular discourse that was scientifically inspired but related to spirituality and religion. Foremost in this group were the Shakers, who by eschewing sexuality entirely made it a central and obsessive feature of their religion—if only by default. And more directly, we see this sexual obsession emphasized in the Oneida Community of upstate New York, which developed sexual union into a religious act of communion. Founded by John Humphrey Noyes in the mid-nineteenth century, the group was progressive, socialist, and devoted to scientific advances as part of a Christian philosophy. The members embraced communal marriage in which the participants were expected to have sexual intercourse with each other. Noyes, like some other "free love" advocates, wanted to separate the sexual impulse from the procreative impulse. For some physiologists, the way to separate these yoked impulses was to use birth control by mechanical means. But many people felt that birth control of this type was unhealthful for the male and female. Thus, for the Oneidans, withdrawal was the rule in all sexual encounters. Females were encouraged to have orgasms, while men were to engage in sexuality but learn self-control through "male continence." Because the community saw itself as a socialist-scientific experiment, debates about the healthfulness of withholding semen were held on a regular basis with external and internal experts holding forth. Some doctors testified that withholding of semen was dangerous while others thought it actually healthful. Only later in the history of the community were selected couples chosen on a eugenic basis and allowed to have children. But the focus of the community, while on religion and industry, was forever bound up with its central sexual message. These arguments were part of an ongoing obsession with and norming of sexuality.

Later, in the beginning of the twentieth century, the mechanics of sexuality continued to be a central area of cultural and social obsession. The book *Karezza* by Alice B. Stockham, a physician and spiritualist, went through many editions. Its popularity is a little hard to understand, considering that it emphasized the virtues of withholding seed. As Stockham notes, "The sexual union which is planned and controlled, becomes glorified through conscious appropriation."[13] The obsession of the period was in the plan and control of sexuality, the attention to the act, and a rigorous set of protocols about how best to do it. As Stockham notes, "The act of copulation . . . is the outgrowth of the expression of love, and is at the same time completely under the control of the will" (23). Using karezza, a couple can avoid "the ordinary hasty spasmodic method of cohabitation" which is "deleterious both physically and spiritually" and instead "through the power of will, and loving thoughts, the crisis is not reached, but a complete control by both husband and wife is maintained throughout the entire relation" (23–24). This withholding of orgasm requires "thoughtful preparation, even for several days previous to the union" (24). Training involves kindly acts, reading, and meditation. Books recommended include those by Browning, Emerson, and Edward Carpenter, a sexologist—an interesting mix of the literary and the medical.

Like the Oneidans, the advocates of karezza used science to maintain the virtue of the practice. Stockham notes that physicians "have demonstrated with incontrovertible facts that it is eminently healthy to conserve the virile principle. The seminal secretion has a wonderful imminent value and if retained is absorbed into the system and adds enormously to man's magnetic, mental and spiritual force" (43). This assurance is added to when Stockham includes a quote from Noyes's pamphlet *Male Continence*. Noyes says that for a man to practice male continence during sexual intercourse is like a helmsman steering a boat in a stream.

> The situation may be compared to a stream in three conditions, viz., 1. a fall; 2. a course of rapids above the fall; and 3. still water above the rapids. The skillful boatman may choose whether he will remain in the still water, or venture more or less down the rapids, or run his boat over the fall. But there is a point on the verge of the fall where he has no control over his course; and just above that there is a point where he will have to struggle with the current in a way which will give his nerves a severe trial, even though he may escape the fall. (121–22)

This navigational analogy is followed by the statement "You have now our whole theory. It consists in analyzing sexual intercourse" (122). It is safe to say that a book addressed to a male reader that recommended the analysis of sexual intercourse would have been impossible even fifty years earlier. The notion that sexuality requires analysis, study, and training—that it is an act that is heavily studied by medical experts who make specific and compelling regulations—is wholly a product of a culture of obsession and connects nicely to the analytic methods of both Zola and Freud.

Thus it was in the first decade of the twentieth century that the words "sexology" and "sexologist" entered the English language, following on the heels of these researchers' efforts. Sexologists began writing books for the general public.[14]

Popular books appeared that translated the science of sexuality, and often eugenics, into practical advice. The stated aim of these books was to provide information for the education of an "ignorant" public. The information often came from progressive authors—often feminists. But the actual process by which these works operated produced somewhat less than progressive results in the long run. In fact, they contributed to establishing rigid norms of behavior and moving sexuality over into a medical category that required medical knowledge, even on the part of the layman, to complete sexual intercourse successfully. Obsessive sexuality as defined by degree, frequency, or choice of object could be established by creating a clear standard of normal, bourgeois, heterosexual activity, often called "married" or "ideal" sexuality.

SEX MANUALS MAKE LOVE COMPULSIVE

One such book typical of this impulse to create categories of normal and excessive sexuality was *Safe Counsel or Practical Eugenics*, which went through thirty-eight editions and sold more than a million copies by 1926. Books like this contained sexual advice, physiological data, often quite detailed charts and diagrams, information on birth control, and general information on marriage, but also popular, amusing, and educational illustrations. For example, *Safe Counsel* advises men against obsessive sexuality, noting that "lust crucifies love." It goes on to say that "sexual excess . . . weakens the vitality, lessens the resistance, and paves the way for many dread diseases."[15] We might imagine that such cautions are a continuation of the expected Victorian morality,[16] but in fact books like these were very much concerned with promoting the advantages and naturalness of sexuality. Sin is replaced by poor hygiene; religious laws and rules governing sexuality give way to medicalized advice on the most effective techniques. *Safe Counsel* finds its core rationale from the moral physiology movement, which linked health and progressive citizenship with the importance of learning "the facts of life." The authors recognize the dangers of sexual continence, pointing out, "[That] sexual abstinence is often harmful we can no longer doubt. The evidence all points that way. The sex instinct is a natural instinct, just like hunger or thirst or fear." But "medical authorities agree that continence up to an age of 25 or 30 years is absolutely harmless. The excess energy is passed off in natural ways assisted by the more active energetic life of the period." Using a "scientific" notion of the nerves as energized or enervated, the book goes on to note that "after maturity, however, the system demands sexual satisfaction. If such satisfaction is not possible, the sexual organs in many instances actually shrivel up. . . . Thousands of neurasthenic men and women owe their pitiful physical condition to nothing but a failure to satisfy a normal natural instinct." What can be done about this? The authors conclude, "Early marriage seems to be the only workable solution. When the hope of such a marriage is held out to the boys and girls as a reward for a clean life, when sex truths are universally taught and acted, when prophylactic, hygienic and eugenic measures are generally understood, there will be no more sex problems."[17] There is a seamless fit between science, eugenics, and proper sexuality—which is wholesome and pleasant to both partners (heterosexual and married, of course).

NORMAL VERSUS OBSESSIVE SEXUALITY

Another such book, written by a Dutch gynecologist Theodoor Van de Velde, is *Ideal Marriage: Its Physiology and Technique,* published in 1926 and translated into English in 1930. The book advocates a "vigorous and harmonious sex life" as the cornerstone of every marriage.[18] To that end, there are detailed descriptions of human sexual anatomy, medical illustrations, graphs and charts—and even more detailed explanations for the proper way to have "communion," or sexual intercourse. After reading this particular book, a layman (and its intended reader is male) would have as much anatomical knowledge as a medical practitioner.[19] The author makes it clear that for a man to have an "ideal marriage" he must master every aspect of gynecological knowledge. The book is frank and open about sexual matters, and it became a much-read and republished work.

Van de Velde promotes a strong notion of a norm in sexuality. He writes:

> I deal throughout this book with such emotions and sensations as lie within the limits of *normal sexuality:* limits which are wide and various enough in all conscience! Morbid deflections, twisted and abnormal desires have no place in the physiology of marriage, in spite of their primitive ramifications, manifold diversity, and extraordinary frequency in the whole field of sexual life. And ideal marriage should be kept free of their taint, with all the knowledge and power at our command. "The pathology of love is a hell whose gate should not be opened at all," says Remy de Gourmont. And we shall be ever careful to keep those sinister portals closed.[20]

Despite a warning about those sinister portals of what Van de Velde might call abnormal sexuality, he does make clear that these non-normal occurrences are widespread. So the line he tries to establish between normal sex and abnormal sex is typically hard to manage. Take his definition: "By 'sexual intercourse,' unqualified by any adjectives, we refer *exclusively to normal intercourse between opposite sexes.* If we cannot avoid occasional reference to certain abnormal sexual practices, *we shall emphatically state that they are abnormal.* But this will only occur very seldom, for, as postulated above, it is our intention to keep the Hell-gate of the Real of Sexual Perversions firmly closed" (144). But in developing this strong notion of normal heterosexuality (homosexuality, by definition, being a perversion), the author has to add that "Ideal Marriage permits normal, physiological activities the fullest scope, in all desirable and delectable ways; these we shall envisage, without any prudery, but *with deepest reverence for true chastity*" (144). So included in acceptable practices are some that others at the time might have considered abnormal, including fellatio and cunnilingus, sex bites, deep kissing, and even some version of light bondage activities.

How hard it is to draw the line between normal and abnormal, despite the heroic efforts of Van de Velde shows up in a discussion of "the normal love bite" (156). He begins saying that "when the love-play culminates and the greatest possible intensity of feeling *is expressed in kisses, both partners tend to use their teeth, and in so doing there is naught abnormal, morbid or per-*

verse" (156). The "normal love bite is an atavistic urge" that takes over during the sex act. Women "are more addicted to love-bites than are men. It is not at all unusual for a woman of passionate nature to leave a memento of sexual union on the man's shoulder" (158). Likewise a man may well grip and squeeze his beloved so that "blue marks of bruises on women's arms are witnesses of the man's '*tourbillion*'" (158). And then there is the "triumphant slap with the open hand on the nates which many a man either gives his partner, or feels an impulse to give her, at the conclusion of coitus." He adds, "these manifestations are quite 'normal,' both in the sense of frequency and of fundamental unconscious motives" (162).

But what goes beyond the pale of normality into obsession? Van de Velde suggests specifically the love bite that breaks the skin and draws blood. Is this normal? "Up to a certain degree—yes. But then there comes a limit beyond which lies—pathological and perverted sexuality. And yet it is very difficult to decide exactly where this border-line lies. As in all departments of emotional life, the stages from the normal to the morbid, from the intense to the bizarre are so gradual that they can hardly be delimited by any hard and fast frontier" (157). He goes on to speculate that every lover is "as one of unsound mind," and then almost cries out in desperation, it seems: "And yet there must be some rule, some guiding sign, some boundary!" (157). This line for him is pain and cruelty, which defines a limit for ideal marriage. However, even that boundary is questioned in his long quotation from Havelock Ellis's "Love and Pain" postulating the desire of the man to inflict pain on his female sexual partner as a remnant of primitive courtship held in check by "the normal, well-balanced and well-conditioned man" (159). And once that check is eliminated, Ellis continues, "when the normal man inflicts, or feels the impulse to inflict, some degree of physical pain on the woman he loves, he can scarcely be said to be moved by cruelty" (159). So Van de Velde concludes that "what both man and woman, driven by obscure primitive urges, wish to feel in the sexual act, is the essential force of *maleness,* which expresses itself in a sort of violent and absolute *possession* of the woman. And so both of them can and do exult in a certain degree of male aggression and dominance— whether actual or apparent—which proclaims this essential force" (159). In this sense, maleness is the sign and meaning of passionate sex, best understood as a violent attack and possession of the female. Obsessive sexuality, then, is built into male sexuality and fully realized in sexual intercourse.[21]

What we see here is a strong need to come up with a sexual norm so that an abnormal, obsessive sexuality can be described and most often delimited. But this attempt is fraught, since so little is known about the varieties of sexual experience. Van de Velde has trouble establishing how much force is "normal." Since he acknowledges the primitive nature of sexuality—and here we have to stop and observe the sheer power of Darwin's and Freud's influence—sexuality is part of the animal, the id, and therefore by definition must be primitive and brutal. The animal is, in fact, male sexuality.[22] How can this primitive urge be controlled and rectified by putting it into the category of the normal? And what is one to do with deviations from this norm? As a contemporary researcher asserts of erotomania, it is "a *construct,* a secular conceptual mirror on which successive views of love, sex and mental disorder are reflected. . . . Views on the rational, emotional and ethical boundaries of love and sex change *pari passu* with whatever image of man happens to be in fashion; 'science' is just another subsystem of the latter."[23] In this sense, the desire to create sexual norms so that abnormal behavior can be defined is at bottom a cultural act more than a rational one.

NORMAL SEX: A USER'S MANUAL

Other marriage manuals, like Helena Wright's *The Sex Factor in Marriage,* published in 1930, are much more programmatic in their relation of science to sexuality. Rather than use physiology as a guide to the body, the author becomes very specific about what to do and how to do it. "It has been discovered that in the majority of women the most complete response follows if they are stimulated in a definite sequence." The sequence is presented as invariable because "these areas seem to be related to one another, so that if the order of stimulation is followed, the response becomes more and more ardent."[24] Many of the works during this period focus on how to bring a woman to orgasm. In this sense, there is a valuable educational principle at work, and the writers of such books universally decry the general ignorance concerning sexual matters. But it is also clear that the attention to the physiology of female sexuality and the virtual ignoring of the mechanism of male sexuality, except in some very general sense of the man's learning to restrain himself during the woman's arousal, contributes to a kind of user manual of the female body. The aim here, as elsewhere, is to establish norms of corporeality, agreed-upon procedures to elicit the orgasm, and templates of normal, heterosexual behavior. The dominant issues of establishing normality by setting limits on quantity, frequency, and kind are presumed to be obvious, and the goal of eliciting the female orgasm becomes a kind of crude benchmark of success, particularly as the orgasm becomes the gold standard for reproduction, health, and mental stability. Obviously excessive sexuality or obsessive sexuality has little or no place in married love, since it would violate the templates for erotic encounters and unbalance the healthful aspects of sexual union.

Books like these marriage manuals develop a scientific attitude toward sexuality that culminates in the notion that one cannot really have sex unless one is properly educated and disciplined in the subject of sexuality. Another way of seeing this is that a norm is developed, based on scientific knowledge, that describes what is the right kind of sex and what is the right way to achieve that sexuality. The norming of sex, and thus the defining of excessive or obsessive sexuality, is accomplished by creating a bell curve of sexuality. For example, Marie Stopes, in her much republished *Married Love,* deflects criticism of her book coming from "some one into whose hands this book falls [who] may protest that he or she has never felt the fundamental yearning" for sexual intercourse. In that case "it is possible that all unconsciously he may be suffering from a real malady—sex anaesthesia. This is the name given to an inherent coldness. . . ."[25]

In this sense, Stopes defines one pole of "normal" sexuality—the profoundly unobsessed person. But her vision of normality in sexual relations is actually one in which most people do not have or enjoy much sexual activity. As she writes, "Leaving out of account '*femme incomprises*' and all the innumerable neurotic, super-sensitive, and slightly abnormal people, it still remains an astonishing and tragic fact that *so* large a proportion of marriages lose their early bloom and are to some extent unhappy" (11). This unhappiness is due to sexual difficulties, which here seem to be the rule in a normal marriage. Stopes envisions disparities between a "strongly sexed husband" who is married to a "wife whose vitality is so low" she only wants sex once a month (62). Stopes's goal is "mutual adjustment"—a compromise between men claiming their "marital rights" and women dutifully submitting. But the net result is a calculus of sexuality, including detailed charts of when a woman is sexually receptive. What we see is a fascinating combination of feminist attitudes citing a woman's right to sexual pleasure combined with a normalizing imperative revealed in statements like the following: "The supreme law for husbands is: Remember that each act of union must be tenderly wooed for and won, and that no union should ever take place unless the woman also desires it and is made physically ready for it. (See p. 67.)" (65). The combination of progressive language and handbook precision ("See p. 67"!) is repeated throughout, as in "This mutual orgasm is extremely important (see also p. 84)" (73). Like other handbooks, this one has strong recommendations that create a should/must approach to sexuality. Stopes speaks of a couple: "Neither he nor she knew that women should have an orgasm. . . . Yet, to have had a moderate number of orgasms at some time at least, is a necessity for the full development of a woman's health and all her powers" (82). So the issue of frequency, intensity, and kind becomes through these books finely tuned to a benchmark of universal moderation.

Normality here as elsewhere becomes problematic because men are perceived as wanting sex more than women do[26] and reaching orgasm more quickly than women. So in the excessive-sexuality model, the solution is one in which men need to practice restraint. The restraint has to do with frequency and with speed. "The husband who so restrains himself, even if it is hard to do it, will generally find that he is a thousandfold repaid. . . . *It should never be forgotten that without the discipline of self-control there is no lasting delight in erotic feeling.*"[27] Thus restraining obsessive and excessive desire for sexuality should be the goal of any happy couple.

It is worth noting that Freud's emphasis on the sexual genesis of neurosis is merely part of a zeitgeist reflected in these marriage manuals. The requirement that women have orgasms is highlighted because, as Stopes points out, "many of the 'nervous breakdowns' and neurotic tendencies of the modern woman could be directly traced to the partial stimulation of sexual intercourse without its normal completion which is so prevalent in modern marriages" (90). As sexuality becomes health, its extremes become pathological. "Thus the ascetic and the profligate . . . have both to run the gauntlet of disease" (107).

MALE SEXUALITY AS OBSESSIVE SEXUALITY

Many of these marriage manuals contain a central paradigm. Normal sex leads to a happy marriage and mental stability. Abnormal sexuality leads to an unhappy marriage and mental illness, particularly for women. But male sexuality, itself, untutored by marriage manuals, is obsessive and in this sense abnormal. Men come easily to sex and need no awakening. "A very important difference between men and women is that men upon attaining sexual maturity in early adolescence uniformly come into full possession of their sexual capacities and do not require sexual experience for the development of these powers."[28] Stopes describes male sexuality as one that "knows no season . . . is always present, ever ready to wake at the lightest call, and often so spontaneously insistent as to require perpetual conscious repression."[29] Thus, husbands, in full possession of their sexual capacities, sexually aroused easily, and left to their own devices, will mount their wives whenever the urge strikes, claiming their marital rights, and will orgasm in a few thrusts. By doing this they will fail to arouse the dormant but present desire in women. Women need to learn sexuality from their husbands, because "in many women desire is very slight until developed by repeated stimulations and experiences."[30] But since husbands follow their natural instincts rather than consulting science, they fail to bring their wives to orgasm and thus create a state of abnormal sexuality. "In most of these cases, the conditions of intercourse have been abnormal through the absence of the appropriate psychological details, frequently because of the dense ignorance of the husband."[31] When this happens, women fall mentally ill. Given the psychophysiological genesis of hysteria and neurasthenia, lack of sexual completion will leave a wife nervous, sleepless, and ultimately hysterical, neurotic, or worse. So the contradiction between the normal, excessive sexuality of the man and the abnormal sexuality it engenders in the woman leaves the sexologists who write and readers who consume these manuals in a state of puzzlement.

The provisional answer to this dilemma is that men must adjust themselves to their wives' periodicity. Thus the normal obsessive nature of men's sexuality has to be tempered to the cyclical desire of women. As Exner notes of this dilemma: "*It is a problem which must be solved* if continued happiness is to be assured . . . This is a compromise, to be sure, but life is full of compromises."[32]

This model of sexual regulation, based on liberal notions and progressive attitudes, has shifted and changed a bit during the twentieth century, but it has never really left the proscriptive model. Even contemporary women's and men's magazines contain the required sexual advice section with specific recommendations to achieve success. Thus obsessive sexuality is proscribed on an individual basis but required on a cultural basis. What this means is that obsessive sexuality is seen as dangerous to marriage, to women, and to bourgeois respectability but becomes a cultural desideratum for society at large. Individuals are condemned for excessive sexuality, but the cultural requirement demands an ecstatic sex life wrapped up in bourgeois monogamy. Obsessive sexuality in its romantic incarnation is found in a variety of literary texts, from *Romeo and Juliet* to *Wuthering Heights* and *Gone with the Wind.* In those works, characters are drawn to each other in a mad and passionate love that is both consuming and ultimately tragic. The moral lesson is that obsessive passion is both a desirable and a dangerous thing.

It is interesting that detailed description of obsessive sex enters the cultural sensorium only in the 1930s with James Joyce's *Ulysses,* which describes in detail the feelings, if not exactly the actions, of furtive masturbation in public and female orgasms. D. H. Lawrence's *Lady Chatterley's Lover* is probably the first semi-mass-market book to describe in some detail sexual intercourse and anal sex. While pornography had been widely available from the eighteenth century on, those works were not generally circulated in bookstores and libraries. The works of the Marquis de Sade or Leopold von Sacher-Masoch were geared to a specific reader of sexual works and were not conceived of as part of a general literary offering. Even so-called risqué works of French writers like Zola and the Goncourts, while they showed us prostitutes and the demimonde, did not attempt to describe in detail sexual acts. The anonymous memoir *My Secret Life* (1902) was a detailed view into a Victorian upper-class man's sexual life, but it hardly was a culturally sanctioned book. It was largely through a cultural process of the inclusion of sexuality into ordinary life, through marriage manuals and through the dissemination of the insights of psychiatry, particularly the popularization of the work of Freud, that narrative scripts of what sex should or might look like developed. As we will see, these scripts may well be linked intimately to the development of current notions of obsessive sex. Through the media and through scientific discourse, an algebra of normativity with various formulas will emerge that place obsession within a negative and positive set of possibilities.

While Freud is enormously important in the discussion of sexuality, it is worth noting that he is not especially crucial in establishing sexual norms. Freud is well known for his theories concerning vaginal orgasms and heterosexuality, but he also recognized, along with his contemporaries, the existence of clitoral orgasms, and his general predisposition was toward seeing humans as bisexual. What is worth noting in this discussion is that Freud was against the notion of a defining norm, particularly in sexuality. He decries, in his essay on Little Hans, "the adherents of 'the normal person,'" who for him are equated with eugenicists and those worrying about degeneration and hereditary taints. Freud goes on to say "that no sharp line can be drawn between 'neurotic' and 'normal' people — whether children or adults" (*SE* 10:141, 145–46). And elsewhere he notes that "some perverse trait or other is seldom absent from the sexual life of normal people" (16:322). For Freud, sexual behavior might cover a range, and whether that range is normal or not is less important than what it tells us about the person or his or her milieu.

RESEARCHING SEXUALITY: A NEW OBSESSION

The proscriptive phase of sexology, which sought to define and prescribe the degree, frequency, and kind of sexuality, gave way to its descriptive phase. Sexologists like Alfred Kinsey, who interviewed thousands of people, and William Masters and Virginia Johnson, who amassed data on over ten thousand orgasms, collectively observed, recorded, and provided statistical norms. While Kinsey was against the idea that morality could assign a certain sexual behavior with the status of being normal, he was in his scientific rigor willing to see what might be statistically normal.[33] Masters and Johnson begin their *Human Sexual Response* citing an earlier call for science to establish "the normal usages and medial standards of mankind" in sexuality and the requirements that "we ourselves issue succinct statistics and physiologic summaries of what we find to be average and believe to be normal."[34] A new tyranny arose as a statistical norm was enforced. If the average length of the erect penis was 5.9 inches and the average frequency of sexual intercourse of married couples was 2.5 times per week, the public now felt the need to measure up, as it were, to the norms. If heterosexuality were a statistical norm, how would that determine one's behavior? Books like M. J. Exner's *The Sexual Side of Marriage,* published in 1938, began using the statistics from sexologists to shape the normal and the abnormal. But of course statistics can often cover the fact that what is being polled is largely culturally determined. So *Facts of Life and Love for Teenagers* from 1950 provides, following this descriptive mode, a flatly descriptive view of homosexuality. "In every community of any size there are men who desire contact with other men and boys. Some of these men actively seek sexual outlets with each other and with younger boys." But this seeming neutral statement quickly leads to the warning, "It is not unusual for a teen-age boy to have been approached in a too friendly fashion by an older man some time in his experience."[35] The author notes descriptively, "Thus we see what might be considered a scale of homosexuality-heterosexuality. . . . In between is the large number of persons of both sexes who at some time in their lives and to some extent find their own sex appealing, but whose capacities for responding to the other sex are also well developed." The answer here is that while it may be normal to feel same-sex attraction while growing up, as Kinsey by now had shown to be common, "its overt forms are not to be actively sought" (89). The reason to avoid homosexuality is that "when this condition becomes chronic, that person is unable to fall in love, get married, and lead a normal life as a man or woman usually does" (271). So, although sexologists of the period may use description as their method, it is hard for many of them to avoid having moral, medical, and cultural norms creep in as a new form of sexual control. Thus the statistically abnormal, the new obsessiveness based on statistical frequency, degree, or kind, replaces the proscriptive or prescriptive boundaries.

Where moral and cultural norms are downplayed, as in Lois Pemberton's 1948 *The Stork Didn't Bring You!*, a "sex education for teenagers," there are biostatistical norms. Under the heading of "homosexuality," Pemberton writes, "Should some glandular deficiency or disturbance exist or arise to cause an over-production of the male hormones in the female body, or vice versa, then we have this condition known as homosexuality."[36] So normal and abnormal are a matter of hormone levels, and therefore the science of endocrinology will enable the "homosexual to resume more normal living patterns."[37]

In fact, even with the science of Masters and Johnson and others, it is virtually impossible to define what constitutes normal sexual behavior. Physiology isn't destiny. One popular book, published in 1947, was Eustace Chesser's *Love without Fear.* Chesser, a British doctor, described on the cover of the Signet paperback as "the foremost authority of sex technique," spends a good deal of time on the question of normality, and even cites Van de Velde. Chesser writes, "For those who are normal, the best way in which to guard against becoming addicted to perverted practices is to develop normal erotic technique to the full. It bestows pleasure which cannot be approached by any abnormal intercourse."[38] He adds, "Normality, too, is the best safeguard against loss of virility."[39] Here we see the emergence of sexuality as a technique, a learnable set of behaviors that can be mastered by anyone who wishes to avoid addiction to perversion. The techniques are by definition "normal," and they produce "happiness" and of course "virility."

A mere five years after Masters and Johnson's work, between 3,500 and 5,000 sex clinics and treatment centers were up and running.[40] Sexology went from research to practice, and sex books based on the research were regular bestsellers. These books offered to increase sexual potency and pleasure and treat what Janice Irvine calls "disorders of desire." These disorders would fall into the hypo- or hyper- areas of disease—from not enough desire to too much, from slow sexual response to too rapid. In fact, a new sexual disease came into being in the *DSM-III:* inhibition of sexual desire (ISD), listed under sexual dysfunctions and considered a mental disorder. It still remains the case that excessive sex isn't listed in the *DSM* while decreased desire is. In this sense, the bedrock measures and practices that would determine what was normal and what was abnormal, what was excessive and what was below par, were in play and in confused play at that.

SEX BECOMES ADDICTIVE

In our own time, sexuality is seen as a good in and of itself. Health and happiness are concomitant benefits, and the issue of choice and negotiation between consenting adults is the norm. The old questions—how many times a day, week, month seem fairly banal. Which orifice, which genital, which person—all have become open to discussion and acceptance. Fetishistic and sadomasochistic practices have become somewhat mainstream, with their own code of morality and behavior (safe words, scripts, etc.). Sexual toys, bondage equipment, and erotic clothing are now available in suburban shopping malls. As a number of sex researchers indicate, we have shifted from a morality-of-sexuality discussion to a supermarket of sexual choices and a language of negotiation. According to the National Sex Forum, established in California in 1968, "As long as people know what they are doing, feel good about it, and don't harm others, anything goes."[41] No longer is anything wrong in sexual relations, as long as whatever one desires is negotiated to the satisfaction of the participants.[42] The only problem is low libido, and even that can be treated with drugs.

Given this free-market approach to sexuality, aided and abetted by the growth of the Internet,[43] sexuality is still not without its governing mechanisms. In response to the efflorescence of sexual choices, a new obsessive category has been created—the sex addict.

"Sexual addiction" is a relatively new term that reconceptualizes the issues of degree, frequency, and kind. A sex addict is someone who is too interested in sex, has it too much, and often with the wrong kind of people—notably prostitutes, other sex addicts, or other sex workers. Of course, in the language of addiction, the problem is not so much the behavior per se or the morality of it, but how you feel about it. If you feel shame or guilt, feel as if the behavior is taking over your life, and so on, then you are an addict. But of course, the "how you feel about it" approach is far from an individual matter. As with OCD, the issue of whether the behavior causes "marked distress" becomes a defining feature of the disorder, without much attention paid to the social and cultural environment. One's feelings of shame and guilt are deeply dependent on the social milieu that defines acceptable and unacceptable behaviors, however openly or subtly. As we have seen, even supposedly neutral guides and articles inevitably contain definitions of normal and abnormal sexuality. Addiction, as a concept, allows for this rebirth of the regulatory mechanisms we have seen earlier, but presents the problem as one of self-regulation, not exterior control—behavior rather than morality or criminality.

To understand how this new regulatory system arose, we need to follow the development of the concept of addiction, a variation on another kind of obsession. The term "addiction" begins to be used in the sense of being addicted to drugs or other substances in the twentieth century. People in the nineteenth century had a range of opiates, barbiturates, stimulants, and other drugs available to them without regulation or prescription. Anthony Giddens asserts that in a traditional society, where one's behavior is socially determined, there is no concept of addiction; but in a society based on individual lifestyle choices, the idea of addiction arises.[44] In fact, it is most likely that many of our grandparents or great-grandparents were addicted to a variety of substances through the use of patent medicines, easily available through local stores, peddlers, and pharmacies. Available opiates included the overused "gripe water," a tincture of opium that helped calm fussy babies. Regulation of drugs occurred in the United States during Prohibition, when people turned from alcohol, then difficult to find, to unregulated marijuana, opium, cocaine, heroin, and barbiturates. The state's response was that if alcohol were banned, surely drugs should follow.[45] The concept of addiction arose in tandem with the criminalization of drugs in the 1920s and early 1930s.

Sexual addiction, as a concept, arose as a concomitant to the twelve-step program for alcoholics, which itself began in 1936 with Alcoholics Anonymous. The twelve-step message entered English-speaking public awareness through word of mouth and a number of significant films from the 1940s through the early 1960s, including *Lost Weekend* (1945), *Come Fill the Cup* (1951), *Come Back, Little Sheba* (1952), *Something to Live For* (1952), *I'll Cry Tomorrow* (1955), *The Voice in the Mirror* (1958), and *Days of Wine and Roses* (1962).

With alcoholism as a medical problem well established by the 1950s and 1960s, we first start seeing books on sexual addiction in the 1970s. Once the idea had been assimilated that alcoholism wasn't a sin or moral failing but simply a physiological problem, a form of chemical dependence predicated on the proclivity of some people in the population to be hypersusceptible to alcohol or other chemicals, then you could move swiftly, on to other "addictive" behaviors like work or sex. By the 1990s, with brain science advancing, the notion switches to one in which people might be addicted not to particular drugs or activities but to the neurotransmitters involved in addiction—endorphins, norepinephrine, dopamine, serotonin, and oxytocin. Just as alcoholics or drug abusers became dependent on their particular form of chemical, so would sex addicts become dependent on their own biochemistry.

Indeed, there was a general ideological trend during this period to remove the onus of moral judgment from certain lifestyle behaviors by seeing them largely as medical problems. Medical discourse, in its elaboration of the concept of disease, moved human activities like obsession from the religious sphere, first to the psychodynamic and then to the biochemical, neuroscientific sphere.[46] People no longer have problems; their brains do.

Yet sexual addiction is caught between medical, moral, and psychological definitions. Further, since it is not listed in the *DSM-IV TR,* it is not an officially recognized psychiatric disorder. Sexual addiction hovers between a popular interest in obsessive behavior and a clinical suspicion of calling something as normal as sex an addictive substance. So, as we will see, the problem is that sexual addiction is not an agreed-upon disease entity. Since it began with twelve-step programs, its origin is distinctly nonmedical. It was only after the idea of sexual addiction permeated the media that we begin to see practitioners playing catch-up.

Because of this heterogeneous origin, there are various and even conflicting definitions of addiction. One writer points out that addiction is "a psychic state that often predates the addict's first encounter with his drug and that remains unchanged throughout the career of his substance abuse."[47] Another writes, "The addict is a person who never learns to come to grips with his world, and who therefore seeks stability and reassurance through some repeated, ritualized activity. . . . The true addict progresses into a monomania."[48] The Web site of Sex and Love Addicts Anonymous (www.slaafws.org), the major organization dealing with this problem, contains the following information: "Addiction can take many forms, including but not limited to, a compulsive need for sex, extreme dependency on one person (or many), and/or a chronic preoccupation with romance, intrigue, and fantasy. Sex and love addiction may also take the form of anorexia, a compulsive avoidance of giving or receiving social, sexual, or emotional nourishment."[49]

One of the immediate questions that arises is, can we say that addiction to sex is a valid form of addiction? The addiction, according to one school of thought, is to one's own biochemistry. Can we say that happy people are addicted to serotonin or sad people addicted to the lack of serotonin? Can we say that nursing mothers are addicted to oxytocin or prolactin or that athletes are endorphin addicts? As one book puts it, "Addiction has as much to do with love as it does with drugs. Many of us are addicts, only we don't know it. We turn to each other out of the same needs that drive some people to drink and others to heroin. And this kind of addiction is just as self-destructive as—and a lot more common than—those other kinds."[50]

Giddens, taking a sociological approach, sees addiction as a function of a society that encourages identity through choice. Rather than favoring Foucault's repressive hypothesis, Giddens proposes the notion that society is reactive to discursive control, creating new options and knowledges. In this sense he is taking his cue from Jean Baudrillard rather than Theodor Adorno, seeing late modernity as based on reception rather than production, tactics of managing power rather than passive victimization by power. So what Giddens calls "institutional reflexivity" creates a society based on endless choices in which "any pattern or habit can become an addiction."[51] Since choice becomes central, addiction then is defined as the inability to choose—you do something over and over again because you can't choose to stop, because you are compelled to perform and re-perform, or think and rethink. In this way, obsession is not about what you are doing, it is about the fact that you can't stop doing it. And the not-being-able-to-stop is finally about losing the much-valued centerpiece of modern possessive individualism—the ability to choose among a variety of consumer options.

But how do we define the sex addict as opposed to any other addict? The direction of Kinsey, Masters and Johnson, and other sex researchers of the 1950s and 1960s was largely a descriptive one. The trend continued through the 1980s so that one researcher could write, "It hardly needs to be said that there is no fixed standard as to how often is too often in sex, whether in terms of total orgasmic frequency, masturbation frequency, copulatory frequency with or without orgasm, homosexual or hetero-sexual frequency, or number of partners. The range of variations is wide, from extreme apathy and erotic inertia to a plurality of orgasms on a daily basis."[52] This distanced observation presented along with the phrase "it hardly needs to be said" reflects the generality of the claim that you can't insist on a norm for sexual behavior, and the only norm is that there is wide variation. Here, as with early sexologists like Van de Velde, attempts to establish a norm for sexual behavior often crash on the shoals of one's own criteria. So if you can't have a norm, how can you describe the point at which normal becomes obsessive, at which sexual activity becomes addic-tion? Since one doesn't choose one's sexual proclivities, all sexual desires are to some degree fetishistic.[53] Why does one person get aroused by one part of the body and another by a different part? Why does clothing or shoes or Italian food or the smell of cinnamon buns call forth desire in some, while the very same things can blunt desire in others?

THE CASANOVA COMPLEX

Indeed, at the very time that the previous rather neutral, nonjudgmental definition of sexuality was written, the contrary moralized notion embed-ded in the language of sexual addiction was arising in popular culture. Pe-ter Trachtenberg in 1988 describes what he calls "the Casanova Complex" as the "compulsive" addiction of men to multiple partners. Rather than accepting the previous distanced and scientific description of human sexual variation, Trachtenberg is distinctly moralistic. To write his book,

Trachtenberg interviewed about fifty men whom he found by placing classified ads. He wanted to speak to men "whose relations with women were characterized by brevity, instability, and infidelity."[54] By boning up on psychiatric and psychoanalytic literature and having discussions with experts in the field, the author prepares himself for his task and ends up saying, of these men, "Their happiness seemed strained and self-willed . . . one encounters an underlying hunger and impoverishment of spirit and an unconscious view of women as faceless instruments of pleasure, ego gratification and relief" (19). By calling their condition a "compulsion," Trachtenberg emphasizes, "I have implied that Casanovas are sick people" (29). The author offers, at the end of his book "options available to Casanovas who wish to achieve 'sexual sobriety'" (21). Concomitant with a language of description, a language of proscription is still very much alive. And as with many of the popular books on sex addiction, the author is not a doctor or a researcher, but a writer with some smattering of knowledge in the field. The twelve-step approach encourages a kind of contemporary version of nineteenth-century amateurism or enthusiasm in which self-examination and very general social observations are enough to draw rather large conclusions.

Obviously, there is a difference between the sexological and the twelve-step, self-help approach. But the difference I want to point to more clearly is that once sexual activity is framed as a disease or addiction, it moves from the realm of a neutral descriptive narrative to another kind of recuperative narrative. The broadly used concept of sexual addiction resides in some interstitial space between science and culture. Because sexual addiction is not in the *DSM-IV TR,* to many that would mean that it isn't clearly a psychiatric disorder, and therefore really isn't a disorder. What interests me is the legitimation, the evolution, of sexual addiction as a category of illness that arose through a popular twelve-step movement and that became, or is becoming, a quasi-clinical entity. How does such a movement happen?

One way to think this movement through is to consider the history. Since Trachtenberg uses the name of the famous lover Casanova, it might make sense to look back to the eighteenth-century man who gave his name to sexual addiction. Reading through the memoirs of Giacomo Casanova and their reception one notices a complete absence of any medical notion of sexuality. The earliest reference to Casanova in print was written in 1823, the same year the book was published in German.

Countess d'Albany writes, "Have you read, Madame, the Memoires of Casa Nuova? It is a book worse than the *Confessions* of Rousseau, but an observer and philosopher can make discoveries there not to be made elsewhere. One cannot understand how an old man of seventy could write such a confession without blushing and without remorse. He makes me detest both men and women at the same time."[55] While there is certainly a note of moral concern, there is no sense that Casanova had a medical or a psychological problem, monomania, let alone a complex. Heinrich Heine mentioned the memoirs in a letter composed in July 1822, saying that "an autobiography stirs up much interest here." In describing the book, Heine writes, "I would not recommend it to a woman I cherish but would to all my male friends. Out of this book there emerges a breath of sultry Italian sensuality. . . . There is not one line in the book which is in harmony with my sentiments but there is also not one line which I did not read with pleasure."[56] By 1835 another writer ranks Casanova's sexuality and his interest in learning along with that of Rousseau: "Equally thorough and learned in voluptuousness and science, such is the motto I would place under the portrait of this Jean-Jacques who, without doubt, was the most remarkable figure in the social life of his century." That same writer sheds possible light on how some viewed Casanova's sexuality, noting that "a questionable mock modesty of our century has rejected his *Memoirs* with moralizings, and the police have come to the aid of this prudery by forbidding, in this or that German State, the most remarkable of all books."[57] Another commentator in 1851 mentions that Casanova is "one of the most original adventurers of the eighteenth century" and that his book is "valuable for a knowledge of the customs of those days, as well as of history."[58] We can perhaps note that before sexuality emerged as a distinct field of professional knowledge, sexual encounters weren't subject to the categories of normal, abnormal, diseased, or healthy.[59]

ADDICTIVE BOOKS

If we use books like Trachtenberg's as an example, we can see that self-help manuals, popular trade titles, and the like have a very important role in developing social concepts of disease in the twentieth century. Such books, along with journalism and other media, disseminate these concepts through the general public so that ordinary people acquire a language for describing some of the complex and ineffable features of emotional and behavioral life. There is an entire book to be written on this subject, but in this space I'd like to point out that many of the books involve a first-person involvement and often a conversion experience. So Trachtenberg, Caveh Zahedi, who made the movie "I am a Sex Addict," and Michael Ryan, who wrote *Secret Life,* tell their own stories, ending up with salvation or at least the prospect of cure through the twelve-step program.

Works like these, often using scientific sources, studies, and surveys, also rely on composite fictionalized accounts of people who are usually given pseudonyms. As one writer explains his method: "This is in some ways a personal book. . . . As the book has broadened in scope, I have developed the theme wherever possible in the form of psychological vignettes. These are fictional accounts, inspired not so much by clinical observations as by normal experience. Although fictional, the characters in these accounts are in a sense familiar to us all."[60] Another writer laments the absence of psychological studies and research, saying "We are aware that we are jumping ahead of research by describing as clearly as could be what we have gleaned from our personal and clinical experiences."[61] Such books are not designed to operate exclusively in the realm of the factual, but rather they work in the area of the ideological, the imagined, the narrativized. People become types; behavior loses any ambiguity and becomes clear and knowable. Although a veneer of scientism permeates the work, there is also an underlying armature of moralizing. We read sentences like "[Addiction] is a malignant outgrowth, an extreme, unhealthy manifestation, of normal human inclinations."[62]

FROM GOD TO PSYCHOLOGY TO BRAIN CHEMISTRY

There is a link between this kind of moralizing and the twelve-step programs, which require the acknowledgment of a "higher power." While all programs stress that the higher power doesn't have to be God—it can be nature or the universe or even the group itself—the God model dominates many of these books, as it does in the conclusion of Pia Mellody's book when she says, "We have found that with the help of a higher power, whom we call God, we *can* stand the pain of reality."[63] God turns up in the handbook to Sex and Love Addicts Anonymous where participants are told that a "reliance on God or some other source of power beyond one's own resources" is necessary.[64] And although the non-God alternative is permitted, the rest of the handbook simply expresses thoughts like "And it is here that true love, which is of God . . . is found and expressed."[65] My point here is not that one should or shouldn't believe in God, but that a quasi-religious and thus moralistic approach is embedded in the sex-addiction program. In that sense, it is a continuation of the proscriptive and prescriptive lesson plans developed by progressive and forward-thinking people.

In this development of a sexually addicted personality, there is a dance of explanatory systems. Is the problem of psychological origin? Is it a problem of chemical addiction to certain neurotransmitters that are produced during sexual arousal? Or is the problem simply one of addiction in general? Stanton Peele claimed in 1977 that "addiction is not a chemical reaction. Addiction is an experience—one which grows out of an individual's routinized subject response to something that has special meaning for him—something, anything, that he finds so safe and reassuring that he cannot be without it. If we want to come to terms with addiction, we have to stop blaming drugs and start looking at people."[66] This language points in several directions—toward a "people-first" way of thinking that gave us "people with disabilities," "people of color," and so on. The aim of Peele's book in the mid-1970s was to take "constructive steps toward a more flexible, people-centered definition of addiction" (49). There is also a demedicalization trend, coming out of the deinstitutionalization movement, and a distinctly behavioral and social model that addiction is conditioned by routine, society, and social pressure. Further, addiction is expanded away from drugs to a wider variety of substances or activities—food, sex, work, and such a wide range of activities that "addiction is not an abnormality in our society. It is not an aberration from the norm; it is itself the norm" (18).

Trachtenberg's book, appearing in the 1980s, hasn't made the complete transition from psychodynamic explanations to chemical-imbalance/neuroscientific models. So he writes, "Like those diseases [alcoholism and drug addiction], it [the Casanova complex] seems to be linked to narcissistic disturbances in early childhood."[67]

It is also worth speculating that at least two of the three major hallmarks of the 1960s—sex, drugs, and rock 'n' roll—have in the 1970s become problems that require care and cure. Peele's book argues that drugs are not inherently or even actually addictive, continuing in a 1960s mode of touting the benefits of certain drugs like marijuana and LSD, while deferring the addiction from drugs to people. In effect, according to Peele, there is no real pharmacological addiction aside from the mental and affective conditioning to the use of drugs. Interestingly, he argues that pharmacologists had already, in effect, agreed to his assertion by changing their emphasis from physical dependence on drugs to "psychic dependence"—a term which Peele rightly notes is so broad and meaningless that it does not apply to a drug per se, but to the mind that becomes dependent on the drugs.

The addiction model for sexual behavior has more recently been perhaps not replaced but refined with a parallel notion of compulsivity. The attempt has been made to bridge the gap between the nonmedical self-help programs and the therapeutically oriented practitioners of sex therapy. Indeed, the major professional journal is called *Sexual Addiction and Compulsivity: The Journal of Treatment and Prevention.* Compulsivity gets the issue out of the demotic twelve-step programs where it began and into the psychiatrist, therapist, and mental-health practitioner's office. Part of this process is no doubt a response to managed health care, the need for diagnosis, and the now ever-present need to use standardized diagnoses developed in the *DSM.* In that direction, compulsivity is now a measurable phenomenon, whereas love addiction was more of a conceptual category.[68] As a clinical entity, compulsivity is defined in terms that hark back to the nineteenth century's definition of monomania: "not being able to choose to engage in the behavior; continuing to engage in the behavior despite negative consequences, and obsession with the behavior."[69] Quantifiable scales were designed to calibrate compulsivity risk-taking, and the researchers who developed these measures concluded that a significant score on risk-taking is predictive of compulsive sexual behavior. Interestingly, this research then cycles into popular magazines like *Glamour.* An article in the June 2006 issue titled "Is There a Casanova Gene?" notes that "guys with a lot of chemical [dopamine] tend to be spontaneous, risk-taking and highly sexual."[70]

But the attempt to recast the nature of sexual addiction from a subject for demotic self-help groups to a professionally treated illness is somewhat fraught because of the difficulty of arriving at the clinical entity. Is abnormally active sexuality an addiction, a compulsion, or actually part of the obsessive-compulsive disorder paradigm? These are partly questions of turf. If you are for the twelve-step model, you'll argue for addiction. If you are a psychologist who uses psychometric scales, you might go for compulsion, and if you are a psychiatrist already familiar with OCD, you

might want to fold the behavior into a known category in the *DSM-IV TR.*
The debate rages on in the professional journals.[71]

BUT WHAT ABOUT LOVE?

Sexology created a science of human sexuality, but there also needed to
be a science or at least a philosophy of love in order to develop a notion
of obsessive, addictive, or compulsive sexuality. Anthony Giddens traces
briefly the rise of romantic love in the nineteenth century and shows how
romantic love sets up a paradigm for romantic narratives about love, essentially separating love from passionate sexuality, now confined to ex-
trarelational affairs and episodic encounters.[72] Marriage manuals of the
twenties through the fifties increasingly substitute the word "love" for the
word "sex." Titles like *Love without Fear* or *The Power to Love* are typical.
And there is also a trend in marriage manuals away from sexual physiology
and toward a glorifying of love as the ultimate rationale for sex. Now we
see sexuality and spirituality joined at the hip (or hips) in reminders like
"lack of physical response tends to loss of spiritual intimacy."[73]

Then, of course, the sixties brought forward not only sex, drugs, and
rock music—but also peace and love. Love was never without its problematics, and Freud and his followers developed a coherent if controversial
knowledge set about love, attachment, and object relations. Indeed much
of psychoanalysis was formed around the specific diagnosis of obsessional
neurosis, ultimately a diagnosis about love gone wrong. So in the fifties
and sixties, notable books like Erich Fromm's *The Art of Loving* developed
models about what love is and should be. Fromm wrote "Is love an art?
Then it requires knowledge and effort."[74] Love is not a spontaneous feeling, a thing you fall into, according to Fromm, but it is something that requires thought, knowledge, care, giving, and respect. And it is something
that is rare and difficult to find in capitalism, which commodifies human
activity. People become couples out of desperation to escape alienation,
a form of teamwork, and do so with a kind of commodified exchange of
"personality packages."[75] Love is corrupted into what Christopher Lasch
later called "a haven in a heartless world."[76] Freud's emphasis on sexuality, according to Fromm, was accurate but misplaced: Freud substituted
sexuality for love and made no clear distinction. Love, for Freud, was a
displacement of the sexual instinct, a translation of nineteenth-century
materialism into psychoanalytic theory. Fromm also critiques Harry

Stack Sullivan's notion of sexual cooperation as merely a cooperation of egos. Fromm focuses on neurotic forms of love—excesses of transference, dependence, poor object relations. He describes "neurotic disturbances in love" in which a person might be fixated obsessively on the mother or father, and so cannot break the obsession and have a "normal" relationship.[77] For Fromm, love isn't something natural. Rather it requires discipline, concentration, patience, faith, and the overcoming of narcissism. It isn't a feeling, it is a practice.[78]

Fromm and others developed a notion of the right kind of love—a normativity of love that was usually coupled with a hypothetical entity called "the healthy couple" or a "healthy relationship." Obsessive sexuality would lie outside of this normative amorous bubble. While Fromm saw love in the context of a political transformation of society and a psychoanalytic perspective, he raised the bar on love from an event that occurs in one's life to a practice and a vocation that required work, thought, and philosophical engagement at a level remote from most people's abilities. This hypostasized and hypothesized love as a state of being is the outcome of a relationship between two emotionally healthy people who are not afraid of intimacy, have not had early problems with attachment and separation, can give and receive love freely, and have a "healthy" sexual relationship, yet are willing to suppress "unhealthy" sexual urges for the greater good of the relationship. Laura Kipnis cleverly ridicules this working at being in love in her book *Against Love.*

Self-help books about the problematics of obsessive love tend to note that a healthy sexual relationship should be predicated on the idea that a couple accept limerance as a temporary state and that a long-term relationship will not have the ardor of a first night or the honeymoon period. The handbook for Sex and Love Addicts Anonymous points out that "the sex and love addict would come to substitute the thrill of sexual adventure or intensity of 'love' for the more encompassing satisfactions, founded first and foremost on self-respect, and later realized in family, career and community."[79] In this scenario, the thrill of sexuality, the lure of ecstatic sex between two people, is supposed to winnow down to the more communal, networked satisfactions of career, marriage, and community. In this account, there is no civilization of discontents, no conflict between eros and psyche. The electrical surge of honeymoon sexuality is supposed to run down to the apparently less distracting and more comforting low-wattage baseline of the domestic space and the workplace. What is essentially a bourgeois vision of life, rife with work-ethic values and utilitarian views of human relations, receives a degree-zero camouflage as simply the right way to live.

CODEPENDENCE AS LOVE ADDICTION

Codependence is part of this scheme, a variation on the addiction scenario added in the 1990s. It too comes directly out of Alcoholics Anonymous, part of a dawning realization that the problem was not solely the addict, but also the family and friends who constitute a network for the alcoholic. This notion is linked to obsession in the sense that the codependent person is fixated on another person for approval, sustenance, and so on. So, for example, in her book *Facing Love Addiction* Pia Mellody can write, "Love addiction, therefore, is an addiction that often becomes visible to the codependent only after some work has been done on the core symptoms of codependence."[80] For Mellody, the Love Addict (her capitalization) is a person who is fixated on another person. She writes "Love Addiction, like other addictive processes, is an obsessive-compulsive process used to relieve or medicate intolerable reality. Caught in the throes of withdrawal pains [when the Avoidance Addict—the other half of the codependency model—pulls away], Love Addicts start obsessing" (27). Here love addiction can lead to sexual addiction, food addiction, drugs, alcohol, and any other variety of elements. These Love Addicts compulsively act out their plans. So in this scheme love addiction leads to obsession and compulsion, although it is not always clear which is the cart and which is the horse. All this addiction is pinned on the expected donkey— early childhood problems. As Mellody writes, "I have come to believe that people fall into love addiction because of unhealed pain from childhood abandonment" (14). Her belief in this etiology seems to be based on her experience as a "nationally recognized authority on codependence" rather than on any professional expertise or research. And this kind of expertise is a problem in the realm of addiction literature. It's worth noting here that I have nothing against self-help programs, and I recognize that many people have been helped by them. But it is also important to note the history, problematics, and contradictions of such a movement, developed piecemeal by nonprofessionals. Indeed, also significant is a recent study that showed that there is no proof that twelve-step programs "are superior to any other intervention in reducing alcohol dependence or alcohol-related problems."[81]

In the eighteenth and nineteenth centuries, as we've seen, obsession developed from doing one thing too much. So the disease and the etiology were the same—you did one thing too much and you ended up obsessed, that is, doing one thing too much. But the addiction scenario has a much less clear arc of causality. Why is one person a sex addict and another not? Mellody's conviction was held by a number of practitioners until the 1990s, when the brain chemistry model began to be accepted. Previously, the unhappy childhood/narcissism model held sway. Craig Nakken distills this insight down to its most commonplace explanation: "There are persons who are more susceptible to addiction. These are persons who don't know how to have healthy relationships and have been taught not to trust in people. This is mainly because of how they were treated by others while growing up, and they never learned how to connect."[82] Here we see the modern mythology of the healthy relationship, the abnormal addict, and the simplified explanation of early childhood etiology. As Nakken notes,

> Addiction is a "pathological relationship." What does this mean? To be pathological is to deviate from a healthy or normal condition. When someone is described as being ill, we mean that this person has moved away from what is considered "normal." The "pathological," therefore, means "abnormal." Consequently, addiction is an abnormal relationship with an object or event. All objects have a normal, socially acceptable function. (10)

Nakken illustrates the modality of addiction-speak: There are obviously normal people who live a natural and healthy life. Then there are addicts who are abnormal and live unhealthy lives. In addition, the world is itself bound up in this fairly obvious natural path of life, controlled, as always, by the famous higher power. As Nakken explains: "With a spiritual Higher Power we learn to perceive and accept a natural order, a natural flow" (22).

STALKING: LOVE ADDICTION WITH A PASSION

Simultaneous with the construction of sex addiction was the formulation of a new category of the obsessive relationship: stalking. The concept of stalking, like that of sexual addiction, arose through social production rather than through medical discourse. Neither sexual addiction nor stalking is found in the *DSM-IV TR*. Stalking is perhaps the next logical development from sexual addiction. If you start with sexual addiction, the model implies that people will come to see that they are addicts through a process of group interaction and self-revelation. Having determined that they fit the sexual addiction profile, they want to change. The stalker, on the other hand, is defined not through his or her own consciousness but through the consciousness of the person who is being stalked. Stalkers aren't going to reflect and realize they are uncomfortable with their behavior.

Another way to see stalking is as a criminal behavior, so defined by the legislatures of many states and by the legal system. Yet the first anti-stalking law was passed in California only as recently as 1990. Britain's first laws were legislated even later. in 1997. In other words, stalking is a relatively new category. As many books on stalking note, "Stalking is an old behavior, but a new crime."[83] This rationale is one we've seen before with sexual addiction, obsessive-compulsive behavior, and virtually any clinically or socially defined pathology. The behavior has been around a long time, but only recently has the clinical name been given to it. Yet this rationale lacks the insight that the process of defining the behavior itself is a function of a complex and highly implicated history. In this case, the relevant history is the one we are tracing—the cumulative, ever-growing body of knowledge on obsession.

Indeed in the past, stalking had been seen as more a part of the romantic project than the criminal one—from the courtly love troubadours, to Dante's pursuit of Beatrice, to Heathcliff's of Cathy, or Fred Astaire's of Ginger Rogers. Not to make light of the real pain that stalkers cause and the violence they may do, we also do need to realize that an obsessed lover's haunting of his object, from Bradley Headstone to Hannibal Lecter, is writ large and often approvingly in the literature of the past and even the present. Obsessive amatory devotion, even unwanted, has been a sign and a token of a deep love that may be desired or envied. Likewise, erotomania in the classical sense, as lovesickness spawned by rejection, was seen as a troublesome but routine part of life. And the spurned lover's attempt to win the rejecter was the stuff of human nature. Recall stalker Helena's desperate plea to her beloved Demetrius in Shakespeare's *Midsummer Night's Dream:*

I am your spaniel; and, Demetrius,
The more you beat me, I will fawn on you:
Use me but as your spaniel, spurn me, strike me,
Neglect me, lose me; only give me leave,
Unworthy as I am, to follow you. (2.i)

Indeed, here we can raise the question, when does behavior move from the social to the medical to the criminal and back again? One can imagine that if Demetrius lived in California now, he might well have gotten a court order against Helena; and she herself might have gone to a therapist or a self-help group for sex addicts or stalkers. It is easy to think I'm being facetious and disrespectful of people who are doing any of the above, but it is a good thought-experiment to see what changes in our view of Shakespeare's comedy if we apply our current way of conceptualizing certain behaviors.

MEDICAL OR CRIMINAL MODEL?

Things get more complicated in the medicalization of criminal acts when, for example, some sexual abusers have wanted to be covered under the Americans with Disabilities Act. After all, they argue, their disease is one that led them to commit crimes. Indeed, given the discourse of sexual addiction, it would seem logical that suffering from an illness could be a mitigating circumstance in a sexual abuse trial. Most recently a young female teacher who had sexual relations with her thirteen-year-old pupil pleaded not guilty on the grounds that she was a sex addict, a position supported by psychiatric witnesses. The confusing thing about the contemporary discourse of obsessive sexuality is that, like the supermarket approach to sexuality—anything can be selected as long as it is done between consenting adults—it is both inclusive and at the same time restrictive. Obsessive studies of human sexual behavior, like stalking, online sexuality, and sex addiction, make it clear that such behavior is part of the variety of human sexual experience. The only thing that makes this behavior cross over into the pathological or the criminal is the amount, intensity, or choice of object. And of course, this fine-tuning is always controlled by some element of social judgment, which itself changes over time.

So the invention of stalking as a criminal behavior, and then a medical one, is part of the general obsessive regulation of obsessive sexuality.[84]

You can see the complex confusion between the medical model and the criminal model in the following statement by Dr. Edward Petch, who in 2000 established a stalking clinic in London.

> The clinic . . . will be designed to assess and manage stalkers and victims of stalking. Given that some of the more intrusive forms of stalking derive from mental disorder, treatment of those disorders may in some cases lead to a reduction in stalking behavior. If the patients attending the clinic did reduce their stalking behavior I would see this as a bonus. The primary objective has got to be the treatment of a psychiatric condition.[85]

How did stalking get to be a criminal activity and then to be proposed as a personality disorder? The activity of stalking involves acts of pursuit of an individual over time; the activity must be threatening and potentially dangerous. Another set of definitions of stalking is

1) a pattern (course or conduct) of behavioral intrusion upon another person that is unwanted;
2) an implicit or explicit threat that is evidenced in the pattern of behavioral intrusion and
3) as a result of these behavioral intrusions, the person who is threatened experiences reasonable fear.[86]

One clinician, J. Reid Malloy, begins the process of converting the popularly and legally arrived at entity of stalking, like sex addiction or addiction in general, into a clinical entity. Malloy makes this move by renaming stalking as "obsessional following." He is aware that the *DSM* definition of OCD involves an activity that is ego-dystonic, that is, an activity or thought that feels alien and unwanted to the self. And he is also aware that for many stalkers their own behavior is not particularly unwanted, at least to themselves. Nevertheless, he argues that the diagnostic term "obsessive" is correct, mainly because the behavior may hover or alternate between wanted and unwanted.[87] Without the authority of the *DSM* (but hopeful of future inclusion), Meloy creates his own *DMS*-like description:

Simple obsessional—based on prior relationship.
Love obsessional—absence of prior relationship.

Erotomaniac—believes self to be loved by victim.

False Victimization—not a victim of a stalker, but wants to be.

In this taxonomy the simple obsessional follower is someone who has had a prior relationship with the victim. The love obsessional is more delusional in the sense that the person has never met the victim, but believes that with due convincing, the person might be encouraged to have a relationship with the pursuer. The erotomaniac is further down the delusional path in that this stalker believes himself or herself to be loved by the victim, although they have never, or only briefly, met. Finally, the false victim is not someone pursued by a stalker at all, but would like to be or believes himself or herself to be. Of all these classifications, only erotomania is listed in the *DSM* under delusional disorders, probably by virtue of its nineteenth-century provenance.

With the coinage of "nymphomania" in the beginning of the nineteenth century, erotomania, as excessive sexuality, quickly became conflated with monomania by Esquirol in 1838, when he wrote that this was "a chronic cerebral disease, characterized by an excessive love for an object either known or imaginary; it is a disease of the imagination and is accompanied by an error of judgment."[88] From the start, there was a problem with Esquirol's definition, which saw the behavior as the symptom of a medical condition. As Berrios and Kennedy put it, Esquirol's definition "was not received favourably by clinicians, who on account of their religious convictions did not want the boundaries between bad and mad to be blurred."[89] Bénédict Morel opposed Esquirol, claiming that "in saying the former [erotomania] is just a disorder of imagination one confuses crime with madness."[90]

EXCESSIVE SEX AS CULTURAL GOAL AND REVILED ACTIVITY

It is clear that this confusion remains to this day. Sexual obsession and excessive sexuality teeter between desired cultural goals and reviled criminal activities. How can Nabokov's *Lolita* remain one of the great books of the twentieth century? It is a book that is revered by many who seem to share a general amnesia, forgetting that lovable Humbert Humbert is in fact a pedophile with horrid aims and methods. Lolita isn't a comely young woman as she is in the films, but rather a twelve-year-old at the beginning of the novel who is "four feet ten inches in one sock."[91] Humbert's desired age range for nymphets is nine to fourteen. His original plan is to drug Lolita and have sex with her unconscious body—not once, but for forty-five drug-induced nights. He masturbates frotteuristically by rubbing against her buttocks and ejaculates as he sits beside her on a couch in the family living room. Humbert, in fact, invokes the dialectic between criminal act and private obsession:

> Ladies and gentlemen of the jury, the majority of sex offenders that hanker for some throbbing, sweet-moaning, physical but not necessarily coital, relation with a girl-child, are innocuous, inadequate, passive, timid strangers who merely ask the community to allow them to pursue their practically harmless, so-called aberrant behavior, their little hot wet private acts of sexual deviation without the police and society cracking down upon them. We are not sex fiends! We do not rape as good soldiers do. We are unhappy, mild, dog-eyed gentlemen.[92]

The popularity of works like *Lolita,* echoed in the late twentieth century by the success of A. M. Homes *The End of Alice,* another story of two pedophiles—one an older man in jail and the other a nineteen-year-old girl with whom he exchanges letters—shows us that deeply embedded in our cultural consciousness is a special place for sexual obsession. Homes's work, which describes sexual abuse and sexual homicide, is touted by *Publishers Weekly* as "a lurid but weirdly arch page-turner" and by *Newsday* as "a provocative exercise in transgressive sexuality."[93] Likewise, Bret Easton Ellis's *American Psycho* and Thomas Harris's *Silence of the Lambs* are novels that are highly acclaimed, have been made into films, and have become part of the American, if not the global, iconography. It is hard to imagine, in fact, contemporary adult narrative without the component of obsessive sexuality. There is an apparent cultural conflict between the scientific notion that sexual behavior is hardwired, requiring medical care, and the legal and moral definition of behavior as worthy of punishment. Recently, films like *Little Children* and *The Woodman* attempt to present stalking pedophiles in a more sympathetic light, showing us characters who are aware that their behavior is abnormal, want to stay in the realm of normality, but struggle with inner instincts.

At the beginning of the twenty-first century, we remain caught between material explanations of excessive behavior and thinking and volitional ones. Much of the twelve-step language, including terms like "enabler," "addict," "codependence," and so on add a moral edge to a notion of volition. If you could just stop addictive sexuality, if you could stop being an enabler, stop being codependent, you could end the cycle of addiction and dependence. But the material explanation now widely available limits this notion. The *New York Times* cites a neuroscientist who says, "To a neuroscientist, you are your brain; nothing causes your behavior other than the operation of your brain."[94] In this argument the free will and self-actualization of the late twentieth century comes to a screeching standstill in front of Vilayanur S. Ramachandran's notion that we don't have free will, we have "free won't."[95] In other words, our brains determine what we do, and all we can try to do is actively stop that forward movement.

In this chapter, we've seen that models for organizing sexual obsession and excess are heavily dependent on particular viewpoints of society at given times. There is, however, a consistent trend of trying to determine what is normal sexuality so that excessive and/or obsessive sexuality can be described and proscribed. Even in ages that seem to endorse a purely descriptive approach to sexuality, the regulatory mechanisms come into clear focus when we look at the edges of what is thought to be normal sexuality. The mechanisms to describe how sexuality is excessive and obsessive are, as we've seen throughout, infused with obsessive attention themselves. Their impulse to describe etiology, diagnosis, and cure remains largely impressionistic and confused. Yet these attempts are taken quite seriously in some circles and continue to provide thriving models for the sexual addict, the stalker, the pedophile, among others—models which themselves enter into the cultural and aesthetic sphere bearing the contradictions of the weak theories that are meant to explain these varieties of human experience.

7

Obsession and Visual Art

Obsession has become collectible. Indeed, the value of an artist increases if the work is seen as the product of obsessive, sometimes life-destroying, angst. The link between genius and obsession is assumed to be commonplace in our own time. But there was a development over time of the link between obsession and value in art. If we turn to two actual visual artists flourishing at the end of the nineteenth century in Germany and Switzerland, we may provide two cultural roadmaps into obsession. In the first case, the obsessive art of Max Klinger, we see precisely an artist whose content and form is obsessive, but whose life is not. In the second case, of Adolf Wölfli, the artist is someone who is institutionalized and his art is seen as the product of his disability. His art is not obsessive, but his life is seen as the product of his disability.

MAX KLINGER'S HALLUCINATORY OBSESSIONS

Klinger, like Monet, was an artist of series—known for his drawings and etching suites, including "Deliverances of Victims Told in Ovid" (thirteen etchings), "Eve and the Future" (six etchings), "Intermezzi" (twelve etchings), "Amor and Psyche" (forty-six) and many others. His best-known series is "Paraphrase on the Finding of a Glove" (ten etchings). One could argue that series painting fits nicely with an obsessive aesthetic, and indeed series paintings coincide with the era of monomania in Europe. In

Klinger's case, many of his works are fantastical, erotic, and bizarre. Repeated elements and animals thread symbolically through the works, although the meaning of the symbolism is elusive. One can argue that this work isn't obsessive, as it is simply a formal exercise. But I want to argue that the elements that bring the series and the repeated image into the aesthetic lexicon may indeed be related to a culture of obsession arising during this period.

"A Glove," made by Klinger when he was twenty-one and his first major series, begins with a view of a skating rink in Berlin with a variety of bourgeois skaters arrayed across the ice. Notable, at least in retrospect, is the artist, perhaps, talking to his friend, who may be contemplating a lovely, young, seated woman. The second etching (fig. 7) shows the young woman's back, canted to the right as she leans into her skating foot, oblivious to a dropped glove, which is retrieved by the Klinger figure as he bends, reaching toward the ice, his own hat fallen down in the process. A group of three skaters tilt toward the left of the painting—emphasizing the overall effect of being off-balance and out of kilter. What follows is a ruminative series of visual hallucinations on the glove. Several show the artist in despair or nightmarish sleep or fantasy over the glove and presumably the woman who lost it. The most famous of these shows a pterodactyl-like creature flying off with the glove as a pair of male hands reach desperately for the purloined object (fig. 8). The surrealistic nature of the picture is enhanced by the impossibility of the image from an aeronautic as well as a zoological point of view.

Likewise, another image of the young man twisting in bed in the midst of a nightmare, his pillow propped up against a Herculean glove while the ocean pounds against the bed and strange sea creatures and a drowning man wash up against his sheets while a pair of hands reach for the man or the glove (fig. 9). What is noteworthy is that the obsession of the artist is clear in the work, is in a way the defining characteristic of the work, and the theme of haunting, repetition, and fetishism needs no explication. We can easily place Klinger in the 1880s when hysteria was being discussed, when Krafft-Ebing's catalog of sexual fetishes and obsession comes to print, and the young Freud was beginning his work with Breuer. But unlike those artists in Zola's work, Klinger is neither mad nor suicidal. His working in series is not seen as a symptom; rather it is the obsessive content of his work that is valued for being so provocative. Unfortunately for the theorists who see obsession as leading to madness, Klinger enjoyed

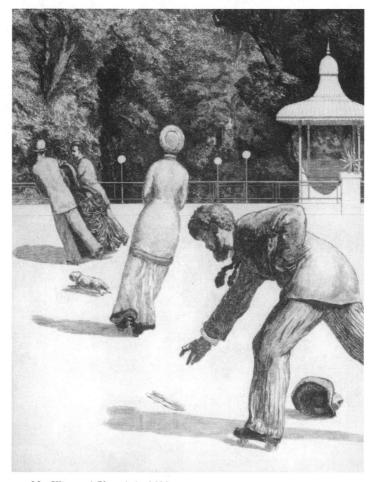

FIGURE 7. Max Klinger, *A Glove: Action* (1881).

the most bourgeois of lives. Far from going insane, he lived rather conventionally, spending his time between Berlin and a country retreat.

Yet Klinger produced a strange and eccentric body of work filled with obsessive themes — death, sex, disease, degeneration. How to think of the art of an obsessed man without thinking of the man as obsessed? Later twentieth-century curators were driven to invent elaborate backstories to link the bourgeois man to the obsessed work. Indeed, the twentieth-century catalogs for Klinger's work and his biographies flail around trying to tie the artist to some kind of pathology. One critic tries to steer the issue to

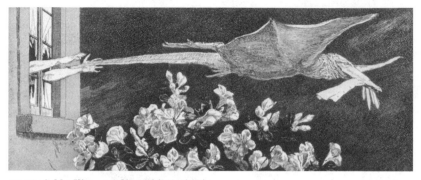

FIGURE 8. Max Klinger, *A Glove: Abduction* (1881).

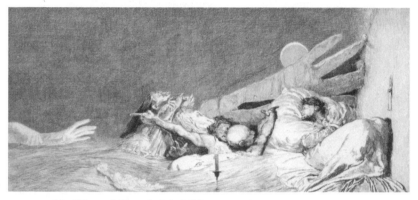

FIGURE 9. Max Klinger, *A Glove: Anxieties* (1881).

the more general: "May be this is not about the madness of love but about the madness of the artist, not Klinger's in particular, but the general lunacy of artistry, which might set a creative or overheated mind in full spin before some emotionally charged object."[1] To bring the psychological to the fore, these critics have had mainly recourse to Freudian analysis of the works. As another critic writes of Klinger's bizarre subject matter, "It might, for example, be seen as evidence of a personal psychological problem, a combination of hypersensitivity and escapist emotional instability. . . . However there is little in Klinger's biography to support such interpretations." The critic mentions that "pathological" explanations fall short, and calls for the same strategy that the previous critic employs — looking at "an aesthetic dilemma affecting numerous European artists of his generation . . . the problems of the modern psyche."[2]

Yet any approach to Klinger that denies the obsession connection, that seeks to see the work as an object, is performing a kind of programmatic reductionism. If Klinger was living in the developing world of psychiatry during a period in which obsessive behavior was being observed, widely commented upon, and included in literature, would it make sense to omit this central point of organization? Could Klinger complexly be refracting the obsessive aesthetic of the time, which shows up in the literary works of Poe, Melville, Balzac, Zola, and others?

ADOLF WÖLFLI: OBSESSIVE OUTSIDER

Another example, this time of a person who was incarcerated in a mental asylum, allows us to consider a work of art from the viewpoint of a more fully developed obsessive aesthetic. Although Adolf Wölfli was an inmate in Waldau Mental Hospital, or perhaps because of that fact, he managed to create an enormous oeuvre comprising over 25,000 pages of writing and drawing before he died in 1930. Of course, simply noting that output will suggest, as many writers about Wölfli do, that his work is obsessive not only in theme and content but in production. Wölfli had a great sense of organization about his work, numbering his pages and sewing the sheets together into books (fig. 10). The obsessive nature of the work is revealed not only in the organization of the material but in the constant repetition of decorative motifs, images, and so on. The work itself is filled with minute, repeated images, words, numbers, and designs (fig. 11). It is always possible to downplay the obsessive nature of this work, as journalist Peter Schjeldahl does when he states: "The common critical deprecation of outsider artists as hermetic obsessives, like birds fated to repeat their single songs, does not apply to Wölfli, whose work is robustly varied and subject to development, however odd. (Come to think of it, many a fine artist has won admission to the modern canon with an obsessive, essentially unchanging manner.)"[3]

But Schjeldahl inadvertently stumbles on the formulation we have been circling around ourselves, that the obsessive in art is deeply involved in the notion of art itself, particularly modern and contemporary art. Given that approach, and the pathological approach, two views of Wölfli and other outsider artists emerge: as artists *because* of their mental condition or as artists *despite* their condition. In either case, the obsessive cat is out of the bag—either pathologized or hypostasized. The obsessive artist is

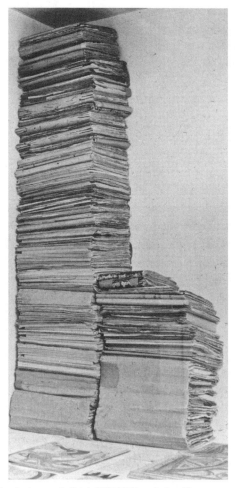

FIGURE 10. Wölfli's books (ca. 1920). © Adolf Wölfli Foundation, Kunstmuseum Bern, Switzerland.

in need of an obsessive audience, and it was only when Dr. Walther Morgenthaler published his *A Mentally Ill Person as Artist* in 1921 that Wölfli came into the critical eye. But Morgenthaler had been watching, detailing, enabling Wölfli to produce his opus since 1907, when the psychiatrist arrived at Waldau. Before that time Wölfli had been limited to two black pencils a week, but Morgenthaler increased the number and provided colored ones. In essence, Wölfli's obsessive work was a coproduction with his obsessive observer—both remembered for the effort put into the output and the reception, and without which the "artist" Wölfli would not

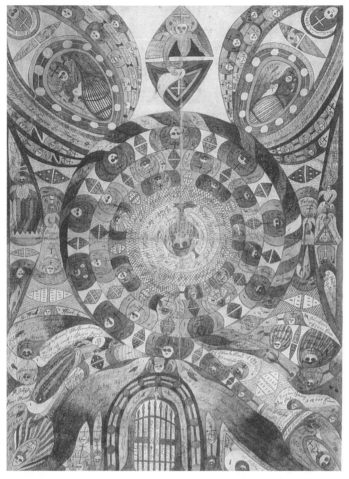

FIGURE 11. Adolf Wölfli, *The Meider-Giant-Cellar in Australia* (1909). Pencil and colored pencil. 99.6 × 72.1 (A9241-6). © Adolf Wölfli Foundation, Kunstmuseum Bern, Switzerland.

have emerged from the inmate whom staff had previously described as scribbling "stupid stuff."[4] It seems clear that Wölfli would have never emerged to public view had obsession not been in the cultural imagination at the time—both regarding the act of creation and the observation of that act. An example of how the lack of obsession on the part of the psychiatric observer can fail to preserve obsessive art can be seen in connection with the following drawing (fig. 12) by a young boy, a piece of art that resembles, in some ways, the work of Wölfli. In this case, the psychiatrist wrote clinically of this drawing, "Even providing unstructured

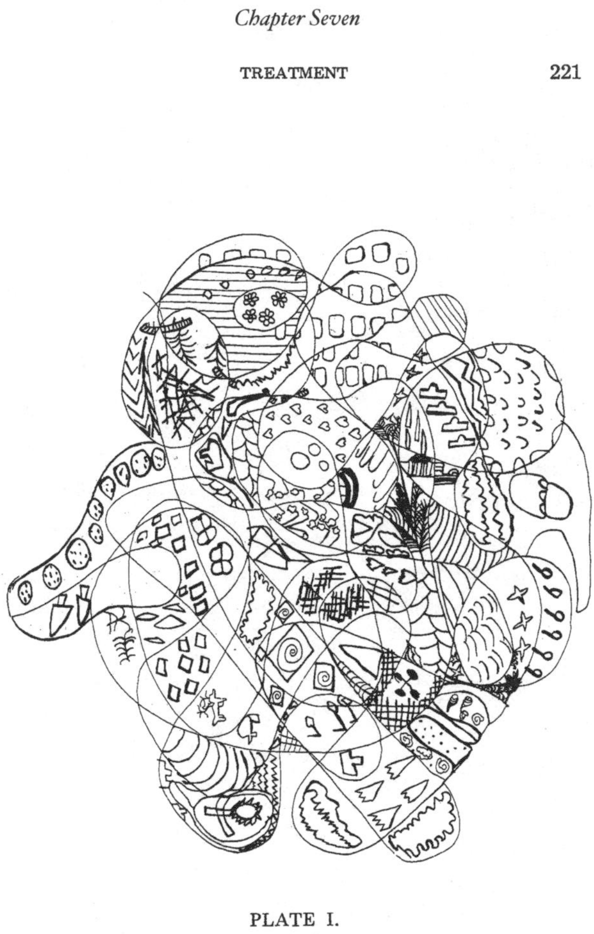

PLATE I.

FIGURE 12. Drawing by child with OCD.

play materials . . . is risky with an obsessive child: he will do time consuming, meticulous and ornate (but not very creative) drawings, such as that
in Plate I."[5]

Unlike this latter-day psychiatrist, the surrealists received Wölfli's work
with great appreciation and the artist was lionized. Later, his work was
seen as one of the prime examples of *art brut*. André Breton called Wölfli's
production "one of the three or four most important oeuvres of the twentieth century."[6] That is a rather grand claim, but it would be repeated for
the obsessive work of the next artist we consider, as if the obsession ups
the ante and the value of the work.

JAY DEFEO: ART AS DOING ONE THING OBSESSIVELY

In the interim from Wölfli to Jay DeFeo, we can track a significant change. Obsession moves from a nexus of pathological surveillance to an existential reason for the value of the artist's work, as it was with Beat generation artist Jay DeFeo's oeuvre *The Rose.* Some half a century after Klinger and Wölfli, DeFeo's work is noteworthy for the way that obsession is imbricated into it. Jay DeFeo was twenty-nine in 1958 when she began the mammoth 128 ⅞ inches by 55 inches work that was to become a foot thick with paint, mica, and wood and that ultimately weighed in at over two thousand pounds. In the introduction to a book on that painting, Marla Prather calls the work "a masterpiece in sheer scale and weight, length of physical evolution, or justifiable mythology."[7] DeFeo worked exclusively on this painting for eight years, and when she completed it in 1966, she stopped painting for three years. In 1958, when DeFeo began, the canvas was much smaller than the finished one, and it was called *The Death Rose.* Later, the smaller work was glued to another, larger canvas as it began its process of growth toward monumentalism.

Her labor was repetitive and endless. Like Penelope working on her loom, DeFeo would scrape away layers of paint and then add more layers. "I sharpened knives on a drill press and hacked and carved the surface," DeFeo noted (42). The fervor and mutilating quality of the technique is reminiscent of Claude Lantier's slashing and gouging of his "masterpiece." Martha Sherrill wrote of *The Rose:* "It was not one painting but as many as five or ten paintings, piled up one upon another" (30). The obsessive nature of the creation also became an accretion to the work. Listen to Sherrill's description:

> The process of its magnificent accretion seemed to consume her. It was as though the work exerted a strange magnetism, pulling everything toward it—people, paint, needles from the Christmas trees in DeFeo's studio, and the artist herself—refusing to let go. It was never-ending. It was both laughable and tragic. People joked that the work would be finished only when the artist herself died, and a myth grew up around them, DeFeo and *The Rose:* a religion, a relationship, a compulsion, an addiction, a fabulous love affair that would not end. . . . For eight years, she worked on little else. (30).

The language around the work recalls the nineteenth century's intense fascination and destruction that such work held for Balzac's Frenhofer and Zola's Lantier. The obsession is now embedded in the object, manifested in the way the work pulls everything toward it in a cynosure of obsession, everything becomes the painting, and the artist is in a way the pawn of the work, chipping away at it, scraping, chiseling, and then layering paint back, like a slave to the compulsivity of the opus.

The canvas was so massive and heavy that it could not easily be removed from DeFeo's studio by conventional means. Two feet of plaster and molding were cut out of the building so the painting could be lowered to a truck on the street below. Experimental filmmaker Bruce Conner shot the event, and his short *The White Rose* became a cult classic. Thus, the obsessivity interwoven into the project was now no longer seen as a pathological symptom, but actually as part of the climate of an event worth recording in another art form—film. A sort of obsessive observation, notation, and documentation follows the obsessive creation, as was the case when Morgenthaler recorded the details of Wölfli's work. The work not only becomes artifact for its formal component, but it develops a special meaning because it is driven by an obsession. In fact, for some years the Conner's film was better known and appreciated than the original painting (33).

Even when *The Rose* arrived at the Pasadena Art Museum, DeFeo could not stop working on it. She felt the painting wasn't ready. The curator of the museum, James Demitrion, observed in DeFeo "a sense of obsession. A huge identification, in a way, she didn't want it seen, as though it would reveal something unseen in her. She wasn't ready to expose herself yet" (31). She spent another three months in the museum reworking the painting.[8] The storage space that housed the work, previously used for a photography exhibition, was painted black and came to be referred to as "the cave." DeFeo's life during the "cave period" began to fall apart. Like the denizens of Plato's cave, she confused reality for images. Barbara Berman, assistant curator at the museum, tried to keep the obsession within a classic romantic narrative: "Losing her painting, her marriage . . . she was in a very fragile state" (31). When the painting was finally exhibited, the paint was eight inches thick in places and was not dry.

The painting itself had a relevant subsequent history that figures into the mythology surrounding it and DeFeo. On moving *The Rose* back from Pasadena to San Francisco, the paint cracked and some chunks fell off. A number of museums expressed interest in the crumbling work, but none wanted to pay for it. Because DeFeo was unwilling to donate the work, the damaged and cracking painting was eventually bolted to the wall of a conference room in the San Francisco Art Institute, where she taught. *The Rose* continued to deteriorate, and when renovations on the floor above threatened the work, DeFeo contacted the conservator in the San Francisco Museum of Art, who suggested the work be shipped to his laboratory for examination and restoration. But because the painting was so massive and already in a state of self-destruction, he suggested an elaborate and expensive plan to take the first steps at preserving the work on site to ready it for the arduous transition. After that *The Rose* would have to be hoisted by a crane from the window of the conference room and shipped to the museum. The painting was thus first covered in a layer of wax, then mulberry tissue, shreds of excelsior, starch paste, and cotton sheeting, and then the entire work was caged in chicken wire onto which was slathered a thousand pounds of plaster. The work was now entombed, returning it eponymously to its earlier name of *The Death Rose*.

At this point DeFeo ran out of money, having paid for the initial preparation herself. Bruce Conner, who had made the film about the painting, tried to raise the needed funds, but in the three years that followed the "completion" of the work, DeFeo's personal life and depression had contributed to a falling-off of her reputation as an artist, and hence of the value of *The Rose*. Now the painting became no longer the work of an obsessive artist but a failed attempt by a discredited artist. The painting lingered entombed in the conference room, encased in the many layers of preservative material, unrecognizable. Institutional memory began to fade. The buried work devolved into an object onto which students put out cigarettes and scrawled graffiti. When the room was used as an exhibition hall for student art, one judge almost gave an award to the housing of plaster, thinking it a minimalist sculpture (33). Eventually, the dirtied object became an eyesore, and the institute put up a fiberboard wall around it, effectively completing the entombment. Somewhere behind layers of wax, paper, chicken wire, and now a false wall, lay the original *Rose*.

Then DeFeo died in 1989 of lung cancer.

How the work was rediscovered and finally restored is painstakingly recalled in the book *Jay DeFeo and "The Rose."* The point I want to make here, however, is that this obscure work finds the light of day not particularly because of some self-evident, intrinsic, artistic value of the work but because of the accompanying narrative of obsession that serves to decode the work. Like a rumor that outlives the scandal, the tale of obsession and compulsion surrounding the work revives the work in its fame and notoriety. Strangely, or perhaps not, corporate and institutional money funds the restoration for the purpose of showcasing the painting in the Whitney Museum's historic "Beat Generation" show in 1995. *The Rose* Conservation Group was formed, detailed plans were made and implemented, and $250,000 was dedicated to the project. The neglected and entombed work had now come to be considered "one of the great masterpieces of postwar American art" (36). Consider just one moment in the process of renovation:

> Inside the McMillan Conference Room, a support structure of two 4,000 pound gantries were assembled, a custom-designed steel carriage frame was set in place, and the painting was lowered onto its face, a tense process that required two days and six professional art handlers. A plywood grid was attached to the painting, and steel pins were embedded into the thickest parts of the paint for reinforcement. Experts were called upon: structural, aeronautical engineers, and consultants from the special-effects studio Industrial Light and Magic, who were specialists in epoxy and fiberglass fillers.
>
> The conservators worked on *The Rose* from the back to the front. Every day they discovered something new. At first it was pockets of air, like tunnels in the paint several inches deep and a couple of inches wide. The conservators filled these with epoxy mixed with chopped fiberglass. They discovered that the thicker areas of paint were quite soft, the consistency of cheese-like clumps. *The Rose* had never entirely dried, and wouldn't for a hundred years. (36)

One is struck by the herculean job of restoration, the time, energy, and devotion that matches the obsession of the creator of the work. In the renovations, however, we see the forces of "rationality," rather than obsession, engaged in a project to exhume and bring back to stability a work which itself is continuously self-destructing, always wet at core, unfinished, changing. No longer is there an issue of personal pathology, only the pathology of the deteriorating painting. The obsession is built into the work, the story of the painting's loss and recovery—all part of the story of art, now a story of various kinds of compulsions.

It is CBS News, instead of an avant-garde filmmaker, who sends a camera crew to document the removal of the painting from the institute. As Martha Sherrill writes, when the work was finally shown at the Whitney it was "no longer a mythical obsession or the albatross that nearly ruined Jay DeFeo . . . no longer mere artifact either. It is a pure experience and a sacred thing, a great work of art" (37). Transformation complete. Walter Hopps, former curator of the Pasadena Art Museum, wrote, "I don't know any other artist in my lifetime who devoted so many years to one work. Few artworks demonstrate such single-minded intensity as *The Rose*" (see fig. 13). Hopps now sees the obsession built into the making of the painting as a measurable standard against which other artists will have to be gauged. How long did it take to make your work of art? Genius becomes, as Thomas Edison had predicted, equally about perspiration as well as inspiration.

While DeFeo's work stands as a monument to her obsession, the work itself is also in the mode of an obsessive aesthetic. Its lines all radiate from a central point. Everything in the painting draws toward the center, as a monomania. The design is geometrical and even somewhat childish, reminiscent of the kinds of easily learned designs one could make with a ruler while sitting in class. The texture and materials have a kind of sameness, too. The work is a kind of living cynosure or whirlpool that pulls everything to its central, idée fixe. In figure 13, DeFeo herself seems to be pulled into the center of the work, a victim in a hurricane pulled toward the eye.

MARK LOMBARDI AND THE OBSESSION OF THE NETWORK

Mark Lombardi's work has no centers of this sort, but rather networks of lines that meander in and out. If the whole story of DeFeo's work is about the centrality of things, the obsession with a core that pulls everything in like a black hole, Lombardi's drawings are rhizomatic, to use Gilles Deleuze and Félix Guattari's term for a type of organization based on decentered root systems like those of tubers.[9]

Lombardi became obsessed with the circuitous way that money flows through the corporate, business, and political worlds. His drawings comprise a compulsively laid out series of circles and connecting arcing lines detailing names, amounts of money, and above all interrelations between individuals, corporations, and politicians or political entities. If all the connections had not been carefully researched, the work could be the ma-

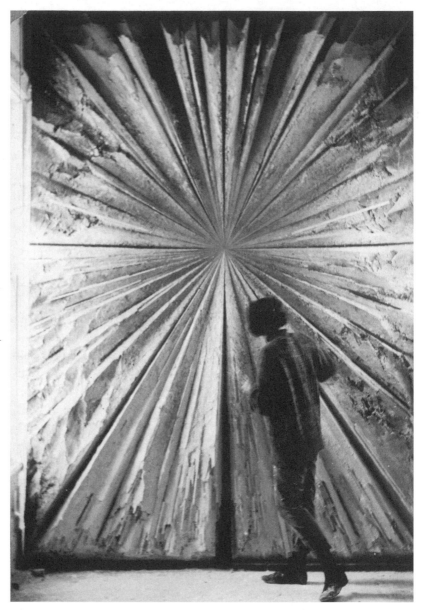

FIGURE 13. Jay De Feo working on *The Rose* (ca. 1960–61). Photo by Bruce Conner, courtesy of the Bancroft Library, University of California, Berkeley.

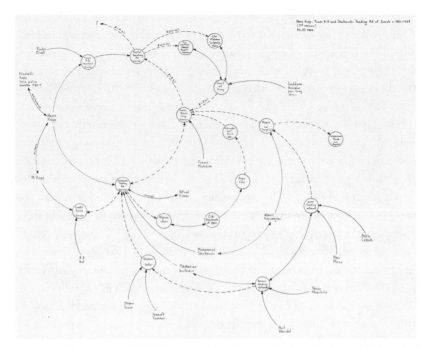

FIGURE 14. Mark Lombardi, "Bill Clinton, the Lippo Group, and Jackson Stephens of Little Rock, Arkansas" (1999). Collection of Mr. and Mrs. Michael Scott. Photo by John Berens.

niacal charts of an obsessive conspiracy theorist. And even the fact that they are researched doesn't eliminate that possibility. These pencil drawings are simply, or rather flatly, presented as flowcharts of power, money, and influence (fig. 14).

As art, the works have value as objects of information. They are visual descriptions of power and money as these flow, in symbols, along a page. But the work is unimaginable without a backstory that is both about the nature of that power and about the motive for visual representation. It seems hard to make a purely descriptive statement about the work without a consideration of motives—on the part of both the names represented and the representer.

At forty-three, in 1994, Lombardi began a series of drawings he called *Narrative Structures*. He had not been an artist of note before this project. Rather he was an art historian, curator, librarian, and writer who occasionally made art. With this project, Lombardi became a kind of amateur sleuth who read newspapers and best-selling books on breaking stories.

Lombardi's tendency was to see connections, conspiracies. He began his major research by looking into the drug policy of the Reagan administration. From this web of crime, money, and politics he branched out into the savings and loan scandals, particularly as they were articulated in the muckraking news articles written by Pete Brewton in the *Houston Post* and then published as *The Mafia, CIA, and George Bush: Corruption, Greed and Abuse of Power in the Nation's Highest Office.* Like the Kennedy assassination, the S and L scandal had many tendrils, and conspiracy buffs have had a field day with them. Lombardi followed this route. His writings on the subject were private, eccentric, and ignored by the wider world. But to aid his researches, he developed flowcharts that helped him map the divagations of money and power. These, it occurred to him slowly, were spectacles and artworks in and of themselves.

The flowchart concept has its origin in several aspects of obsessive behavior. When the Iran-Contra scandal occurred, in which Reagan administration officials were implicated in a complex deal to sell drugs to finance weapons sales to the Contras in Nicaragua, Lombardi followed this new scandal and conspiracy. Ironically, he may have gotten his idea for such a flowchart from a document that Oliver North scrawled to describe his money-laundering through offshore banks. In any case, the writer of his major catalog sees one obsession within another. According to Lombardi, "I was talking on the phone one day with Leonard Gumport, an attorney in Los Angeles, about the outcome of the bankruptcy of Adnan Khashoggi, the Saudi commercial agent and playboy arms dealer who had figured prominently in the Iran-Contra affair. . . . As Gumport spoke, I began taking notes, then started sketching out a simple tree chart, showing the breakdown of Khashoggi's American holdings. Within days, I began making more of these charts, depicting other corporate networks I had researched."[10]

In this case, an obsessive activity leads to the creation of an object that is caught in the crosshairs of that obsessive network and that is then retrospectively inseparable from the obsession that created it. The intricate web of influence and money-laundering that Oliver North spun to finance the sale of arms to the Contras, and even the diagram North made of his plans (fig. 15), came to be the chart of complexity and obsession that launched Lombardi's career.

The catalog for his work, *Mark Lombardi: Global Networks,* begins to use the language we've come now to associate with an aesthetic of obses-

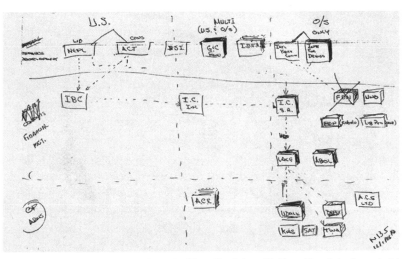

FIGURE 15. The financial flowchart drawn by Oliver North from *The Tower Commission Report* (1987).

sion, noting that Lombardi made "thousands of three-by-five index cards covered with handwritten notations" (16). The actual number was over fourteen thousand (51). The catalog dutifully reproduces a photograph not of his art but of some of Lombardi's index cards and a file box (fig. 16) as a testimony to the detailed and time-consuming work that went into producing the drawings, just as Wölfli's art is buttressed by the photograph of his work piled up neatly into a towering monument. The index card photo then becomes itself part of the performance of the art.

The constructed biographical self and its obsessive activity which produced the work now mediate the value of the art. The catalog also includes telephone interviews with Lombardi's friends, one of whom characterized him as "consumed," "intense," and "frenetic" (17n16). Another says, "He was funny and manic with a racing mind that was always trying to connect the dots. He seemed a perpetual student of interdisciplinary studies" (115). The profile emerges of someone not unlike Lee Harvey Oswald and other loner obsessives: "He worked alone on a solitary project, a massive inventory of facts and the challenge of configuring them in a legible fashion, in a small, lonely room; an internal process. . . . If you were willing to listen . . . he could go on for hours" (115–16). Another friend noted, "I have known Mark to work, without sleep, for days at a time. This might suggest a form of mania that is not at all that rare."[11]

The construction of Lombardi as an artist now is linked tightly to his

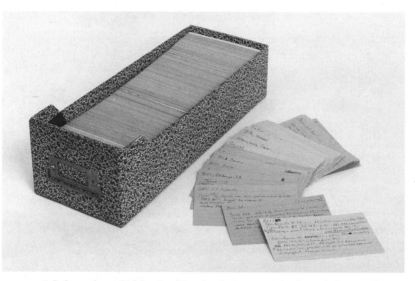

FIGURE 16. Index cards on which Lombardi kept handwritten notes (1998–2001). Courtesy Pierogi and Donald Lombardi. Photo by John Berens.

obsessive research. Ken Johnson wrote in the *New York Times* of Lombardi's "resonant poetry of paranoia."[12] The catalog of his work includes minute descriptions of his working method, implying that it was somehow both rigorous and yet obsessive: "In addition to clipping items from daily newspapers and weekly magazines, Lombardi made extensive lists of government publications and books on particular scandals and individuals, which he then made every attempt to track down. . . . Because many of these publications were out of print, he often asked secondhand book dealers to help him obtain them." This account continues with the inexplicable detail that although Lombardi took materials from the Internet, he wrote everything by hand. "When asked why he had not put this information into computer files, Lombardi repeatedly affirmed the need to write these facts in his own hand."[13] Speculation ensues as to why. This level of discussion, analysis, and observation becomes itself a kind of obsessive disquisition on the nature of Lombardi's compulsive activities. No detail is irrelevant to the ontology of his art.

Lombardi's subsequent suicide by hanging, with the implication that his own studies and drawings were part of a pathological set of paranoid networks that drove him to despair, clinch the narrative convention that links us back to the nineteenth-century accounts of Van Gogh's suicide, an act that pathologizing art critics see as ratifying the work as obsessive, and therefore genius, art. Then a further countercultural narrative develops around Lombardi in which we see the triumph of Reaganomics and the right-wing agenda over the beleaguered artist/activist, with that "explanation" itself becoming part of a feedback loop much like the flowcharts Lombardi had made.

Conspiracy buffs gladly adopted Lombardi, especially after his death. One conspiracy Web site contains the following: "Allegedly diagnosed with bipolar disorder (manic depression), Lombardi supposedly died from suicide (or was suicided) in 1999 — after two successful solo shows and just as his career was about to go to the next level."[14] His pathology is a mark of his artistic abilities, but his death now begins to look like a further act of conspiracy.

Another site says, "The guy put together one chart too many."[15] The one-chart-too-many approach is furthered: "In a video of the artist shown at the exhibition, Andy Mann asked Lombardi in February 1997, 'Do you fear for your life?' Lombardi didn't answer the question. Instead he said, 'This is a way I can map the political and social terrain in which I live.' According to his friends, Lombardi told them that he was being followed — just before his death."[16] A friend writes on a tributary Web site: "When the news of Mark's death arrived, almost all of us thought that he was murdered. We assumed that he had made one too many accusations, and that someone made a phone call."[17] And even more conspiratorially, another Web site says, after describing the suicide of a reporter named Gary Webb, "Gary Webb joins Mark Lombardi, J. H. Hatfield, and Danny Casolaro as the fourth 'suicide' by a researcher who had a detailed understanding of the structure and function of the Bush crime family."[18]

The afterlife of Lombardi attaches his research, his art, his psychopathology, and his obsession to a new link of the conspiracy story. Where DeFeo's work has the single dimension of intense and fatal creation, Lombardi signals, as did his work, a ruminative and obsessive networking, mirrored in his own charts, that links individuals with politics and power in art and in life, which are now inseparable.

JUDITH SCOTT: OUTSIDER INSIDE OBSESSION

Whereas the obsessive nature of the art of DeFeo and Lombardi hovers between the product of an overwhelming desire to make something and the artist's inability to stop doing something, what can we say for artists who do not seem to have the awareness of what they are doing? While this lack of insight may be attributed to outsider artists like Wölfli, of whom psychoanalyst Lou Andreas-Salomé wrote to poet Rainer Maria Rilke that "neither the productive activity nor what it reveals can be held back,"[19] we still can say that with artists like Wölfli there is both intent and awareness. But what about the art of people with affective and cognitive disabilities that limit their awareness of an intentional project.? Of the outsider artist, Fred Tomaselli writes, "I've always thought the sensibilities of 'outsider artists' and Conceptualists were more similar than the art establishment is willing to admit—at their best, they both manifest a compelling and visceral visualization of inner cosmology." This may be an overstatement in search of a reality, but I think Tomaselli's point is helpful for us in thinking about the way that an interior obsession becomes exteriorized.

Can we say that Judith Scott is an obsessive artist? A woman with Down syndrome, Scott could not hear or speak and had no understanding of language. Until her death in 2005 at the age of sixty-three, she had for about sixteen years produced monumental sculptures made out of objects wrapped in twine, string, yarn, paper towels, and other materials. What is clear on viewing her opus is that the repetition of an obsession made and shaped the works. Her method of working evolved. An object was found and wrapped. Scott would work all day for hours on end doing this repetitive activity. She seems to have had no concept of art, sculpture, galleries, or even whether what she did was something that should be started or stopped. There seems to be little of what we might call volition or intention, except in the narrowest sense of the word.

What is interesting is that the very features I have just described are wrapped up with her art. The Creative Growth Gallery Web site, specializing in disabled artists, quotes Scott's biographer and critic John M. MacGregor: "Judith possesses no concept of art, no understanding of its meaning or function. She does not know that she is an artist, nor does she understand that the objects she creates are perceived by others as works of art. Whatever she is doing she is definitely not concerned with the making of art. What then is she doing?"

With Scott's work, and that of other severely impaired artists, we reach a limit in considering obsession—the point at which obsession and severe cognitive impairment collide. Obsession is an activity or a thought array

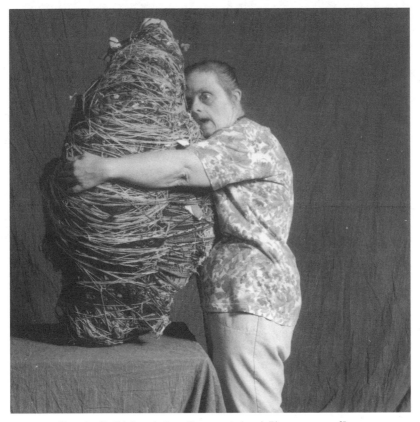

FIGURE 17. Portrait of Judith Scott by Leon Borensztein (1999). Photo courtesy of Leon Borensztein.

in which the subject is doing something or thinking something that will not stop by simple volition. The person is aware of the obsession but is powerless to stop it. With Scott, although the work was repetitive, unending (except by her death), unified around a single concept, it was done without awareness and without the desire to stop. In this sense, the work was mechanical, performed as an automatic activity.

Yet there is an aesthetic, a choice of materials, of design shape, and some sense of desire in the creation of the object. A photograph, whether staged or not, shows Scott embracing her work, as if it were a giant transitional object (fig. 17). The photograph encourages the viewer to see an intimate connection between artist and work, a relationship based on desire. Like Zola's obsessive artist Claude Lantier, the artist loves the work not wisely but too well. Her life is not sacrificed to her work; rather her work gives her life a value. In this case, it is not the obsession that enters the work to create value, but the work itself that creates value in the life of the artist. So in this sense, the work is art not to the artist, but only to the collector. Since Scott attaches no lasting significance to the work of art (she discards each finished work), the repetition abides with the process of creation, not with the object produced. Scott often waves goodbye to her work, as if to signal that the activity of creating is the remainder, while the work is dispensable, a bottle without a note sent out to the ocean.

Can we say that with Scott we come to the end of obsession in art? The repetition, the focus, the helplessness before the process and the desire to return now reaches a point of mechanism. The human motor, as Anson Rabinbach might put it, turns on, but the mind is the motor, not an unwilling passenger. Yet Scott, Lombardi, DeFeo, Wölfli, and Klinger all stand as exhibitions in the hall of obsessive aesthetics.

8

OCD: Now and Forever

Obsessive-compulsive disorder was a rare and strange disease before the 1970s. Estimates for the disorder in the general population at that time were from 0.05 percent to .005 percent.[1] If you were a mental health practitioner, you would expect to see, by the former percentage, one person out of two thousand who had it, or by the latter, one person in every twenty thousand. So in 1973 a researcher could write that OCD was "unquestionably, one of the rarest forms of mental disorders."[2] Consequently, if you were a person with severe symptoms of OCD in the mid-1970s, you would probably assume that you were alone, odd, and certainly crazy. You might even have been treated as someone who fit into the borderline between neurosis and psychosis.

Indeed my own mother-in-law was diagnosed with depression and OCD in the 1940s and was shuttled in and out of mental hospitals, given insulin and electroconvulsive shock treatment, and ultimately diagnosed as having pseudo-neurotic schizophrenia. That diagnosis, no longer used, saw the person presenting as merely neurotic while actually being schizophrenic. There was then an experimental cure for this now nonexistent disease, and that was a brain surgery called a topectomy, no longer performed. So my mother-in-law, in the early 1950s when she was in her thirties, received this operation, in effect a frontal lobotomy, without much effect. She was part of the later notorious Columbia-Greystone project that tried to pioneer psychosurgery to cure mental illness. The project was much hailed initially, and then came under disrepute as the era of psychosurgery finished with a disappointing and brutal close. Her OCD symptoms remained intact until her death some forty years later.

For the latter part of her life, she simply managed her symptoms and never again, understandably, sought psychiatric help. During those years, OCD had gone from a rare and intractable illness, perhaps requiring brain surgery, to a quite common, routinely diagnosed, and treatable disorder. In the meantime the cultural ambient world was peopled with loveable images of OCDers, from Tony Shalhoub playing Monk to Jack Nicholson in *As Good as It Gets.* Most estimates now say that 2 to 3 percent of the population will have OCD during their lifetime; that is two or three out of a hundred people. Recent attempts to describe an OCD spectrum increase the incidence to one in ten.[3]

How did we go from one out of twenty thousand to three out of a hundred to one in ten in less than thirty years? An extremely rare disease has now become rampant. Indeed, the World Health Organization's 2001 mental health report noted, "Four other mental disorders figure in the top 10 causes of disability in the world, namely alcohol abuse, bipolar disorder, schizophrenia and obsessive compulsive disorder."[4] So now OCD is one of the top four mental disorders in the world. Consequently, it has also become one of the most researched disorders.[5]

If you have been following along in the uneven genealogy this book has been presenting, you may well be ready to see that any simple psychiatric definition of OCD or explanation for the uptick in the disorder is bound to be reductionist. It's not simply that scientists are by definition simpleminded, but that medicine tends to want to find "the" single cause for an illness. However, with OCD the explanation can only be complex. This isn't to say that contemporary explanations of OCD aren't complex and even interdisciplinary, but because they inevitably leave out the crucial social, historical, and cultural elements—the biocultural—and fail to examine their own methods, biases, and premises, the explanation provided will necessarily be incomplete.

We have a tendency to assume that professionals and practitioners, particularly if their expertise is in the sciences, have arrived at the definitive concept or idea of a phenomenon.[6] Science, unlike the humanities, discards previous knowledge in place of the most current (and presumably correct) explanation. Yet histories of science and medicine are only optional knowledges for working scientists. So experts in OCD may believe they have little need of the kind of genealogy that I have been presenting. But the complex knowledge my study is offering is not irrelevant, it would seem apparent at this point, to the current definition of a disease entity like OCD. To not very lyrically paraphrase Yeats, how can you know the disease from the history of the disease or the person with OCD from the disorder?

DISEASE OR DISEASE ENTITY?

The first major issue to consider with any in-depth study of OCD is whether the constellation of behaviors and thought patterns that we are calling OCD is a coherent and freestanding one. In other words, are we looking at a disease or a disease entity? I have raised this question along the way, and I would like to consider it again at this point in the argument. In the history relating to OCD, we've seen a number of symptoms and behaviors come and go, be attached and detached, to the constellation of obsessive behaviors. When the *DSM* was first established in 1952 it modified the notion of OCD by separating phobias from obsessions and establishing the obsessive-compulsive personality as distinct from the disorder. In 1968 *DSM-II* codified that distinction between personality and disorder. Each subsequent edition has further modified the criteria for the disease—defining OCD as something separate from schizophrenia or depression; increasing the time required for the diagnosis from three to six weeks; and next perhaps including the idea of an OCD spectrum. Each of these changes makes an alteration to the disease entity, to the number of people who have the illness, and so by extension to the social impact of the disorder.

Have we reached the end of the line now? Are we looking at the cumulative correction of a process of trial and error? Or is the entity we are now calling OCD just as much a disease made by committee as it has been in the past? Michael Stone notes that "no matter how tightly and rigorously we define OCD in contemporary psychiatry, there is still conceptual overlap with various 'diagnostic near-neighbors.'" He notes that it can take on "the coloration of delusion . . . and there is no fine line demarcating *compulsion* from *impulsion* such as to rid these concepts satisfactorily of an overlap." Further, "the common 'fellow-travelers' of OCD (phobia, panic, depression) and the fairly wide range of severity among bona fide cases of OCD will ensure a level of semantic confusion well beyond our day."[7] Another way of saying this is that OCD may not be a discrete entity. One researcher notes that 77 percent of his OCD patients have a lifetime history of another Axis I disorder, while 57 percent who came to a clinic had at least one other Axis I *DSM-III-R* diagnosis.[8] Given the current pitch of research on functional brain activity, neurochemical transactions, and genetic locations, we have to ask if the category OCD is itself something discrete enough to plug into a scientific equation to find the result. For example, if there are likely to be two disorders in the brains of OCD patients, as was just noted, how can any biological test find the single place or problem causing OCD? If there are gradients and continua, how can there be a specific area in the brain with a specific response we are calling OCD? Further, the problem of defining OCD is more difficult in children, where much of what children do is by nature obsessional. As Paul Adams writes, ". . . obsession is everywhere, in all of us. Among children, it characterizes a lifestyle, or a transient and recoverable state, or an unrelenting neurosis, or a severe psychotic illness, or a collective 'game.' Obsessive behavior appears all along a broad and diverse spectrum of childhood activities."[9] It is true that most researchers in OCD will acknowledge that they are always refining and fine-tuning the diagnosis. Currently, it seems, obsessive personality disorder may be removed from the diagnostic manual, and the notion of an "obsessive-compulsive continuum" will be introduced in the *DSM-V.* But is what they are left with a freestanding entity?

If the disease is a structural and chemical disorder, as is argued by current researchers, then, by definition, it can't be a disease that is a result of societal or familial or even individual pressures. That is to say, if you have a broken leg, it doesn't matter to the diagnosis if you are rich or poor, have had a happy or sad childhood, and so on. The extension of that argument is that if you have a broken brain, other factors matter much less as well. To buttress this idea of the inherent and universal nature of OCD, many of the clinical and popular books on the disorder claim that the "illness" has been around since time immemorial. In such books there are only cursory references to 10th-century Persians, Paracelsus, medieval and Renaissance physicians, Lady Macbeth and Dr. Johnson, Catholic Church concerns with religious scrupulosity, and a smattering of other examples. So based on this slimmest of evidence, the claim remains that OCD has always been around and further that it is found in all cultures. Each book that is published—whether clinical or self-help—repeats these snippets of proof in an introductory paragraph or two. Yet the actual historical evidence for the existence of a clinical disease of OCD is scant and would not stand up to scrutiny in a freshman history class. We might want to consider this belief in the historical continuity of OCD as part of an origination myth for those who now work on OCD.

In addition to the "always been around" myth is the putative global nature of OCD "found all over the world." That claim is equally grand although the evidence again is scant, based mainly on the Cross National Epidemiological Study of Canada, Puerto Rico, Germany, Taiwan, Korea and New Zealand which showed OCD to be present in all those countries except Taiwan.[10] Though widely cited, this study is actually a review article that looks at varying data over a rather long period of time in a mere six countries and the US. This hardly represents a survey of the world. A few further epidemiological studies are used to make the global claim. A typical example of how this claim works can be found in a chapter of an influential book on OCD. The author states "The basic types and frequencies of obsessive-compulsive symptoms are consistent across cultures and time."[11] Two footnotes with references are provided. One is a study of the prevalence of OCD in Japan and the other on "preliminary psychiatric observations" in Egypt. Those two articles are the sole basis for the rather sweeping claim that OCD symptoms are consistent across cultures and time!

The epidemiological analyses have been complicated by the fact that "an optimal threshold or diagnostic criterion that reliably distinguishes the clinical from the subthreshold syndrome of OCD has yet to be identified."[12] What this means is that it's hard to identify when the kind of obsessive behaviors that might be part of our culture cross over into a disease entity. A high percentage of the normal population have obsessions and compulsions which are indistinguishable in content from those that are defined as clinical, with frequency and intensity being the distinguishing factors.[13] A standard tool used to determine whether someone has OCD is the Yale-Brown Obsessive Compulsive Scale (Y-BOCS). But with this test, as with any other, a numerical threshold has to be decided, above which you have the disease and below which you don't. In some cases, the cutoff point is a score of 16, but others argue for a cutoff point of 20.[14]

The questionnaire used by the Cross National Study, as another example, seems far from objective:

I want to ask you if you have been bothered by having certain unpleasant thoughts all the time. An example would be the persistent idea that you might harm or kill someone you loved, even though you didn't want to. Have you ever been bothered by that or by any other unpleasant and persistent thought?

- A. Was this only for a short time or was it over a period of several weeks?
- B. Did these thoughts keep coming into your mind no matter how hard you tried to get rid of them?
- Other unpleasant thoughts that keep bothering some people, even when they know they are silly, are that their hands are filthy or have germs on them, no matter how much they wash them, or that relatives who are away have been hurt or killed. Have you ever had any unreasonable thought like that?
- REPEAT A AND B
- How old were you when you first had a problem with this kind of thought or worry?
- How recently have you been bothered by thoughts like this that kept coming back no matter how ridiculous you thought they were?

Some people have problems with feeling that they have to do something over and over again even though they know it is foolish—but they can't resist doing it—like washing their hands again and again or going back several times to be sure they've locked a door or turned off the stove. Have you ever had to do something like that over and over?

Was there a time when you always had to do something—like getting dressed perhaps—in a certain order, and had to start all over again if you got the order wrong?

- Did you have to do this only for a short time, or did you feel you had to do this over a period of several weeks?

Has there ever been a period of several weeks when you felt you had to count something, like the squares in a tile floor, and couldn't resist doing it even when you tried to?

- How old were you when you first had to (do something over and over/check on things/count) do things in a special order?
- How recently have you been bothered by having to do things like this (do something over and over/check on things/count/or do things in a special order)?[15]

I've taken the time to list the complete questionnaire because it seems to cry out for a discourse analysis. The first thing we might want to notice is that the inquirer who asks these questions seems to be leading the interviewee. Rather than simply asking for behavior, the questioner shapes the type of responses, suggests certain kinds of thoughts and behaviors. I've read these questions to a number of people (and I recommend you try it as well), and almost always come up with positive results. In court, this line of questioning would be called "leading the witness." Another feature of the questionnaire, in keeping with our general observations about the dual nature of obsession—a disease to be investigated and a method of investigating—is that the template is repetitive and indeed obsessive, down to the requirement that questions A and B themselves be repeated. The questionnaire groups things together that might not necessarily go together. For example, asking if a person has ever had the idea he or she might harm someone alongside the question of whether they fear that a loved one on a trip might have been hurt or killed is like asking if you've ever eaten chicken or human flesh as if the two things were in the same category. Also the conflating of present and past—(did you have this as a child, and do you have it now?)—creates a mistaken notion of durability over time. The study's failure to distinguish between lifetime prevalence and point prevalence—that is between having something for all of one's life versus having had it at one or two points—weakens the result. It is possible to have been compulsive as a child, in fact fairly normal, and then to worry about certain things or have fixed ideas as an adult. But does that mean there is a lifetime of disease?

Finally, there are methodological issues: this study has been criticized for using nonprofessional, untrained interviewers in some countries. Without highly trained staff, any series of questions like these can be shaped by the tone, voice, and manner of the interviewer, who would clearly be "happy" to get positive answers. Given all this, it's not surprising that this study identified a large number of people as having OCD. Further, how well were the translations of the Y-BOCS checklist tested to assure that they would be standard from language to language? Finally, which groups of people were tested—did they include homeless people, prisoners, the poor? If not, the study itself might tend to reflect the interests of middle-class people and those more likely to be involved in such a study in the first place.

If this seminal study, widely cited, is so full of holes, how can it be used to justify the routine claim of the global universality of OCD? As opposed to this universal existence of OCD, it is possible to make a specific argument about shifting and changing symptoms photographed for a moment in the frame of a concept, itself likely to be displaced at various times. If we buy the latter explanation, then it becomes quite difficult to argue that a specific region of the brain, or a specific arrangement of neurotransmitters, will ultimately be responsible for the occurrence of OCD. You can of course argue that a specific area of the brain may be involved in worrying or planning or checking, but to assume that the brain has a specific location or set of locations for something that itself isn't fixed or universal is a deeply problematic assumption. In other words, if there isn't a locked box that contains OCD and only OCD, then any attempt to find the exact site of something like OCD will be a rather flawed endeavor. It would be like trying to find the place in the brain or the neurochemistry behind the desire to drink a Starbucks latte rather than a Dunkin' Donuts regular.[16]

In arguing for a more complex explanation and understanding of disease entities, I am not saying that attempts to locate the part of the brain in which OCD lives or the chemicals by which it may function are futile endeavors. Indeed, we need to understand the mechanisms of the brain in much better detail, and that prospect is an exciting and complex one. Indeed, more sophisticated analyses of the brain are already ongoing. But I am saying that these investigations are only part of the story, and that the story is not an irrelevant part of the formation of the concept of the disorder itself. When I've presented talks to practitioners and researchers, I see that while many are receptive to, for example, the historical information I bring, they walk away not really believing that knowing the biocultural aura of facts and effects that surround a disease entity has much value in their study of the specific mechanisms, say, of brain function in OCD. If you are trying to find a defective spark plug, knowing the history of the development of the car seems irrelevant at worst and at best merely entertaining. And if you are trying to figure out how the car got to Philadelphia, simply understanding how the spark plug works won't help you. You will need to know the life story of the driver and her current wishes and desires. So what I'm saying is that trying to understand OCD is more like trying to figure out how the car got to Philadelphia, and the approach being taken by researchers is more like trying to figure out how the spark plug functions.

If your model of OCD is that it is based on an imbalance of neurotransmitters or a malfunction of the basal ganglia, a broken-brain model, then you have a static model of the disorder. In that static scenario, you will see the human mechanism as consistently the same—steady throughout all history—and presume that the factors that lead to OCD are distinctly organic and ahistorical, by definition. Environmental factors will be of some interest, but they will generally be seen as universal ones like contracting a strep infection or being exposed to stress.

The universal model will, if the past is any predictor, prove inadequate for a number of reasons. A central one will be that if you locate a brain region, or a neurotransmitter, or a genetic region—or all three—you will still be able to attribute that cause to only a fraction of the total people with OCD. You will then be able to say that 30 percent, for example, of people with OCD have a specific genetic pattern. in a particular gene, but how can you then explain the other percentage that do not?[17] In fact, if the universal, ahistorical notion of a broken brain that needs repair were to be accurate, it would have to describe all sufferers, not a fraction.

In addition, if you adhere to this universal static model, you will have difficulty in explaining why it was that OCD was a relatively rare disease before the 1970s and a relatively common one now. You'll have to say that it was simply underdiagnosed in the past. But that explanation will be evidently inadequate because of the ridiculously dramatic upsurge in numbers—anywhere from a forty-fold to a six-hundred-fold increase. Advocates of the universal model will argue that OCD is by nature easy to conceal.[18] Yet the *DSM* definition emphasizes that the rituals and behaviors characteristic of the disease do not alone define the disease. What really defines it as a disorder is the anguish and "marked distress," the ego-dystonic nature of the beast. And, so it is a diagnostic and conceptual contradiction to say that something that can be easily concealed is to be known diagnostically by a very palpable anguish and despair, not likely, by definition, to be repressed. And then it is also noted that OCD causes great concern and anguish to family members, again indicating that the "easy" concealment argument isn't so easy.[19] I'm not denying that OCD can be kept secret, but that alone cannot explain why suddenly so many more people have OCD.

THE MYTH OF MEDIA EXPOSURE

Another explanation used by many researchers to explain the uptick in numbers is to say that media exposure has allowed people to come forward. When they see OCD on TV, they may identify their behavior and report to physicians that the puzzling things they have been doing have a diagnostic name. There is a lot of truth to the media-exposure theory, but, again, it can't fully explain the forty-to-six-hundred-fold increase in OCD cases. And to the extent that it is true, it is true for many other cognitive and affective disorders, as well. How much of the phenomenon is driven by the very researchers and practitioners who then marvel at the increased numbers?

There is a book to be written following the phenomenon of the development of new lifestyle diseases. Indeed, a general trend toward the medicalization of virtually every emotional and cognitive state is upon us.[20] Within the past fifteen years we've seen ADD, depression, bipolar disorder, insomnia, restless-leg syndrome, sexual dysfunction, social anxiety disorder, and autism, among others, go from either unknown or relatively uncommon occurrences to major illnesses. It isn't the role of this book to document that larger change,[21] but I do want to suggest that the media explanation isn't without its own complexities.

The standard scenario in all these uptick stories is that researchers find a correlation between a certain behavioral/affective structure and a drug or treatment. Studies are done in which a formerly either hopeless or in some cases unknown illness "responds" to the drug or some other treatment. Initially, these studies are wildly optimistic, although few if any are randomized, double-blind studies. Many are in fact done by enthusiastic researchers who are excited about finding a correlation and helping their patients. And let us not forget that careers can be made, funding received, and tenure secured around such successes. In the initial surge of studies on treatment for OCD with Anafranil, a 70 percent improvement rate was cited. And that 70 percent rate was also cited initially for treating depression using SSRIs. Yet there is an inevitable falloff from the initial wildly optimistic accounts. In the course of this enthusiasm, researchers publish their work in journals, and practitioners read the work and give it a try on their patients. TV, print media, and Internet sites tout the cure, inform about the new diagnosis, and people, often family members and friends of the newly afflicted, suggest visits to the doctor's office for diagnosis and treatment. There is a sociology of disease recognition that needs to be developed to account for this phenomenon.

As part of this process, the researchers will mention that the previous regimens were ineffective. The current literature on OCD has a standard narrative that includes the difficulty of treating the disorder, the high failure rate in the past, the poor prognosis, and then the good news of how well the current paradigm is working—not perfect, to be sure, but much more effective. For example, a contemporary researcher will say how bad things were in the past. But were things so bad? The reality of obsession in the past could in fact be substantially different. One researcher in the supposedly benighted 1950s says that 39 percent of the people with OCD showed a good prognosis, while 30 percent did not worsen. So that would be a total of 69 percent who either improved or stayed the same. Another researcher in 1973, citing this work, summarized, "I would suggest that the natural outcome of untreated cases of obsession in childhood is good."[22] So we might want to look with suspicion on how the current moment characterizes the past.

YES, ALSO THE DRUG COMPANIES

Compounded in this process is the involvement of drug companies. David Healy and others have documented how these companies promote their drugs and new diseases by ghostwriting articles to appear in major medical journals as well as providing free video segments for TV stations that appear to be local news stories but serve to promote product and disease recognition.[23] In addition, prominent celebrities with the dysfunction will be hired to appear on national shows like *Oprah* and *Today* to tell their stories. The short take on this complex subject is that pure objectivity is not always part of the process. For example, Dr. Eric Hollander marvels that "in a survey of 701 members of the Obsessive Compulsive Foundation, I found that approximately 25 percent of obsessive-compulsive sufferers first seek treatment after seeing a report in the media about OCD."[24] Hollander seems to take the media exposure as a naturally occurring event, and his own involvement as merely supervisory and helpful. But as is noted in a Medscape interview, "Eric Hollander, MD, has disclosed that he has received grants for clinical research from Abbott, Wyeth, Ortho-McNeil, Pfizer, Lilly, Solvay, and UCB Pharma, as well as grants for educational activities from Abbott, Wyeth, Ortho-McNeil, Pfizer, Lilly, and Solvay. Dr. Hollander has also disclosed that he has served as an advisor or consultant for Abbott, Wyeth, Ortho-McNeil, and Solvay."[25] (Lilly manufactures Prozac; Pfizer makes Zoloft; Solvay produces Luvox, Wyeth makes Effexor—all of which are SSRIs used in the treatment of OCD and recommended by Hollander in his Medscape interview.) While it is not unusual for a clinician or researcher to receive monies from drug companies, it is more than possible that such connections will influence decisions and outcomes, even indirectly. Otherwise, as many people have pointed out, why would these major pharmaceutical companies fund the kind of endeavors they do? The *New York Times* reported in March 2007 that when Minnesota required drug companies to disclose payments to doctors, psychiatrists ranked the highest in such payments, receiving 6.7 million dollars in a single year, with most of the payments going to the few top people in the field who in turn were the most likely to be on professional boards approving the use of drugs for standard practice.[26]

The major researchers in OCD, like any other field, know each other, present their material to each other, appear in each other's books, and meet for committees and professional conferences. While not all agree with each other, most seem to be well-funded by the drug companies that have strong interests in promoting so-called antiobsessional drugs. Michael A. Jenike, who himself has received substantial funding from drug companies, writes, "As the pharmaceutical industry realizes the potential market for effective antiobsessional agents, they are investing millions of dollars in research into new compounds."[27] According to his own Web site, Jenike has received a substantial amount of those dollars.[28] The FDA moved in 2007 to limit to $50,000 the amount of money that an advisor on a drug-approval panel could have received from a pharmaceutical company in a previous year, an indication of how much money is involved in such payments—with the new number being considered a low-end limit.[29]

HIDDEN EPIDEMIC

The print media is a very influential means of reaching the lay public, particularly those publications that public relations experts call "the influencers." Hollander notes that 28 percent of OCD patients came for help as the result of reading, 16 percent from hearing about it on TV or radio.[30] Self-help books on OCD, written by experts or celebrities, bring home the message surrounding the disease entity. These books are always written around a new cure, which the expert touts as the breakthrough that will change things forever.

Most popular books on OCD, and many clinical ones, begin by describing the surge in numbers of people with OCD. For example, Judith Rapoport, whose best-selling book *The Boy Who Couldn't Stop Washing* brought OCD to national prominence in 1989, observes: "The textbooks had told us the disease was very rare. Later we came to see how common the problem really was. . . . [Our] surveys showed that Obsessive-Compulsive Disorder is not at all rare—it is indeed common. Then it quickly became clear that there were treatments that worked. Suddenly, OCD became the psychiatric disease of the 1980s. We began to see many, many patients."[31] This explosion of OCD is also noted by Lee Baer, who wrote in 1991, "When we established the OCD Clinic at Massachusetts General in 1983 . . . I had seen fewer than fifty OCD patients. . . . Since then we have seen almost a thousand, and eight new patients now come to our clinic each week. Our colleagues tell us that similar growth has occurred at other OCD clinics around the country."[32]

The magical narrative in which there are no active agents, merely effects, is repeated here and throughout the tale of OCD. Another book written about ten years later observes that OCD, "previously considered a very rare mental disorder, now appears to be a hidden epidemic. Recent research indicates that over 6.5 million people suffer from OCD, making it one of the most common mental disorders. . . . [OCD] impacts about one adult in 40."[33] The term "hidden epidemic" was echoed in the pages of the *New England Journal of Medicine,* when Jenike wrote his editorial entitled "Obsessive-Compulsive and Related Disorders: A Hidden Epidemic."[34] Hollander repeats the term in his article "Obsessive-Compulsive Disorder: The Hidden Epidemic," in the *Journal of Clinical Psychiatry.*[35] He says "We have overcome the myth that OCD is a rare, untreatable, and psychologically driven disorder" (3). And the title of one self-help book is *Tormenting Thoughts and Secret Rituals: The Hidden Epidemic of Obsessive-Compulsive Disorder.* What exactly is a "hidden epidemic?" It turns out that "hidden epidemic" is virtually a code word used to launch a public relations campaign about a new lifestyle or similar disorder. A casual Google search of the term yielded hidden epidemics for autism, depression, bipolar disorder, sexually transmitted diseases, celiac disease, asthma, chronic fatigue syndrome, hepatitis C, drug addiction, sexual violence, obesity, dissociation disorder, birth defects, heart disease, and, of course, concussion in rugby as well as foot and mouth disease.

If we don't accept the magical forty-to-six-hundred-fold increase in OCD as an agentless process, how can we explain it? One could argue that the old 0.05 percent number might include underreporting, but it also might have included the most intractable and severe cases of OCD. The culture had not yet been fully prepared to medicalize a range of behaviors under the terms of OCD. Let us presume that the researchers were in some sense responsible for the formulating and publicizing of the disorder, and that the swelling numbers followed a pattern typical for the emergence of new disease entities. So the first phase would be the "discovery" of and publications on the disease along with the "new" cures, which seem to be wildly effective. Then there is an inevitable inclusion of people with less severe cases. We have seen this me-too process come about in the example of depression or ADD in which initially only a small percentage of the population saw themselves as fitting the diagnosis, then after a while more and more people consider themselves to fit under the diagnostic rubric.[36] As practitioners become part of the process, people self-identify—with or without the encouragement of friends and family—and practitioners prescribe the medications which the patients themselves know of through the media and often request.

So in the case of OCD could there be a relationship between the relative rarity of the disease and its lack of treatability versus the proliferation of the disease and its somewhat more successful cure rate? The argument could be made that the people who are more treatable are to some extent the newer, less serious cases. One thing that remains a problem for OCD, even with some success, is the rather low rate of cure and the reality that the disorder is chronic. The aim of most practitioners is to reduce the severity and the frequency of symptoms, not to eliminate the disorder, which in many cases seems incurable.

GENETIC, NEUROCHEMICAL, AND OTHER MODELS

Some recent research in OCD indicates there might be a genetic basis for a predisposition to OCD. As with the other work in neurobiology, the aim here is to find a material basis for this disorder. Twin studies and family analyses indicate a correlation between having OCD and having a family member with it. Actual analyses of haplotypes have found some correlation between specific regions of a gene and the likelihood of having OCD. However, even these recent studies come with qualifications and cautions. Since genetic research is increasingly finding that complex disorders like OCD cannot have a single gene or allele responsible for symptoms and behaviors, these studies, very preliminary in their research, must be taken with a grain of salt. As one research group notes, "Family and twin studies suggest that OCD is a complex genetic trait likely resulting from the interaction of multiple genetic variants as well as nongenetic risk factors."[37] And another points out that "no single SNP was significantly associated in both studies. . . . Therefore, to account for these findings, functional variation in this region must be in varying degrees of LD with these SNPs in different populations or multiple functional variants must be present and account for the association with different SNPs."[38] The latter statement indicates that neither of these studies agreed on a single genetic location that would contribute to OCD.

In the rush to explain OCD, researchers rarely note that the various models they use may not fit together very neatly. At least three different streams flow into the neurobiological analysis: chemical, structural, and genetic. But do these streams converge into one larger river? Perhaps not. The standard neurochemical analysis of OCD revolves around the use of SSRIs to treat the disorder. The model claims that there is a brain imbalance of serotonin or problems in the receptor sites for serotonin. When SSRIs correct this imbalance by increasing serotonin, according to this model, then patients improve. As one popular book put it, "Manipulating the body's serotonin levels worked to alleviate OCD symptoms, [so] scientists assumed the cause of OCD must have something to do with this chemical substance."[39]

The serotonin model is well documented and certainly, in regard to depression, seems to be effective (although the actual effectiveness over placebo has fluctuated wildly in studies—with initial studies showing far greater success than later studies, some of which show only a few percentage points over placebo.) Recent research on antidepressants has shown that their initial effectiveness was vastly overrated because pharmaceutical companies suppressed negative results, among other reasons.[40] The new work indicates that SSRIs are only minimally effective over placebo, and in cases where all data was considered, efficacy was not even statistically significant.[41] The problem with the serotonin theory is that. We still do not fully understand how serotonin works in relation to OCD. As Judith Rapoport put it in 1989, "Anafranil probably acts on certain serotonin receptors, but it is still unclear whether the net effect is to increase or decrease serotonin itself."[42] Now it is assumed that there is an increase in serotonin levels in parts of the brain. But how that works to stop obsessions is still unclear. Further, we have no way of actually measuring serotonin in the brains of patients, and can only infer the level of serotonin by measuring it in platelets. This indirect way of measuring is not necessarily accurate. The best way to measure brain levels of serotonin is to directly access the brain, not a procedure most volunteers or patients would agree to. The other problem is that the "imbalance" model implies that there is a level of serotonin that is normal and that imbalances can be calibrated and measured. Yet we cannot say with certainty, for example, that if you have a certain level of serotonin you will be happy and if you have less than that you will be depressed or have OCD. Serotonin levels fluctuate from person to person, and one person with a high level of serotonin may report being depressed while someone with a low level of serotonin might report being happy. Serotonin might help people with OCD because it ultimately will treat their depression—but can that outcome be said to treat the OCD?

Some genetic models indicate that the brain chemical in question is not serotonin, but L-glutamate. Is there a conflict between the serotonin model and the glutamate model? As researchers put it, "The focus on a single receptor or neurotransmitter is undoubtedly a gross oversimplication of a difficult, intriguing clinical problem."[43]

BROKEN BRAIN?

The brain scan model is equally problematic. Clearly parts of our brain are active in various activities. For example, a recent study of brain activity claimed to have located the regions involved in the act of shopping. Knutson et al. have shown that activity in one region will show preference for a product, another will compare prices, and a third will make the decision. In their words, "Distinct circuits anticipate gain and loss, product preference activated the nucleus accumbens (NAcc), while excessive prices activated the insula and deactivated the mesial prefrontal cortex (MPFC) prior to the purchase decision. Activity from each of these regions independently predicted immediately subsequent purchases above and beyond self-report variables."[44] So when we shop, we activate various parts of our brains. When we worry, plan, have anxiety—all activities involved in the disease entity of OCD—we will use various parts of our brain. Will we discover, for example, that the "normal" shopping circuits in our brain are different for people who shop too much? Too little? What will we have shown if we find different or underactivated circuits for shopping? In other words, we have to be careful not to attribute to the brain single locations for activities that are socially determined, constructed, and complex. The human brain did not necessarily evolve to shop, although selecting fruits and berries from among various bushes might well be something we evolved to do. But shopping is not that, and there isn't a place in the brain for shopping. There well may not be a place in the brain for OCD either.

Despite the confidence of various researchers and self-help books, the exact areas of the brain and how they work are not clear. The accepted truism at the moment is that the areas involved in OCD are the right head of the caudate nucleus with orbital cortex and thalamus activity.[45] Benkelfat et al. found a decrease in the normalized left caudate nucleus but not the right.[46] But then another research team has found that the anterior cingulate cortex (ACC) in patients with obsessive-compulsive disorder (OCD) is hyperactive at rest, during symptom provocation, and after commission of errors in cognitive tasks.[47] There still is no agreement on where in the brain OCD resides, although more sophisticated studies on neural pathways are in the works. Several areas have been located, but there are more general questions about whether the brain works in networks rather than locations. That is, whether the areas that metabolize glucose (and thus show up on brain scans) are in fact the place where the activity resides or only one spot of a vast interactive neural network.

As I said earlier, it is vital that we understand the workings of the brain. But there is a larger philosophical question at play. What does it mean to say, in effect, it's all in the brain? If we decide that OCD is based on a broken-brain model, and we can fix that broken brain with drugs or behavioral therapy, then what are the ramifications of this kind of approach? Let's say that we can pinpoint the fact that sexual pleasure is located in a specific part of the brain,[48] or that we ascertain that religious feeling is located in a different part of the brain.[49] Does this mean that we should understand that when we have an orgasm we are essentially having sex in our brains? Or that a religious sentiment is made possible by certain brain functions? Then would someone who does not experience religious bliss have a broken brain? And should we think of Viagra as a brain drug? Will sexual dysfunction now be considered a brain disease?

The implications of the notion that OCD is the result of a broken brain need to be thought through more carefully in the type of research we are seeing. For example, if we could locate the place in the brain where humans feel that killing another human is wrong (some combination of empathy[50] and moral judgment[51]), then why would it not be possible to claim that murderers in fact suffered from brain malfunction and were ipso facto unable to stand trial? This discussion leads to a longer one about free will, which it isn't the goal of this book.[52] But the point I am trying to make is that while it may be relatively easy to find places in the brain that show activity by using PET scans or fMRIs, it is much more complicated to talk about what it means to "have" a disorder; to experience a physical, cognitive, or affective sensation. Our technology perhaps encourages a one-for-one analysis of complex states by showing us specific brain activity. But just because a region lights up on a screen does not mean that this region is itself the state we are examining. We implicate a region in a behavior, but we have so much more explaining to do beyond that "fact." As one brain researcher was reported to have said in a discussion of whether or not there is a place in the brain that governs homosexual desire, "Human sexuality was a complex phenomenon that could not be reduced to interaction of brain structure and hormones."[53]

In describing the creation of the disease entity of OCD and particularly the treatment of the disorder, what we are seeing is a synchretic tendency to move to multiple models and at the same time a resistant drag toward keeping a single, monolithic explanation. The interdisciplinary thrust of the exploration—combining drug regimens with behavioral/cognitive therapy, seeking genetic, neurochemical, and functional explanations—is encouraging, but the default position is the reflex toward finding the single explanation, the specific location, the one drug category that will "solve" the problem of OCD. The reality is that Occam's Razor can be a dangerously blunt instrument, and the simplest cut isn't always the kindest or the best.

SUCCESS NARRATIVES

The explanatory narratives about OCD always concern the issue of treatment. As the uptick story is repeated in each article, essay, or book, so too is the tale of the previous difficulty of treating OCD and the current success, downplayed but nevertheless part of the success story. As the story goes, in the past OCD was a very rare, largely untreatable disorder. Psychoanalysis and psychotherapy were ineffective, although they might provide some limited insight. Then, when drugs like Anafranil and Prozac came along, the largely untreatable and rare disease became both treatable and common.

This is a compelling and attractive story, particularly to the researchers and practitioners who write the articles and books about OCD. It is an attractive story to the people with OCD, who would of course want to champion a cure. But does the story have a basis in history and fact? As I think will become apparent, while scientific papers in journals are scientific insofar as they deal with the collection of data under controlled conditions (in the best experiments), they can be very weak, if not error-laden, when it comes to putting together a narrative, doing history, interpreting data, and so on. The double check on accuracy supposedly comes with peer review, but as recent studies have shown, peer review still leaves many studies vulnerable to error. Indeed, one roundup article in the *Scientist* declared, "Indeed, an abundance of data from a range of journals suggests peer review does little to improve papers." The article goes on:

> In one 1998 experiment designed to test what peer review uncovers, researchers intentionally introduced eight errors into a research paper. More than 200 reviewers identified an average of only two errors. That same year, a paper in the *Annals of Emergency Medicine* showed that reviewers couldn't spot two-thirds of the major errors in a fake manuscript. In July 2005, an article in *JAMA* showed that among recent clinical research articles published in major journals, 16% of the reports showing an intervention was effective were contradicted by later findings, suggesting reviewers may have missed major flaws.[54]

Given the fact that the peer reviewers of articles are often involved in similar research, an inherent bias toward progress and success can be reflected in the review process. And few if any reviewers or researchers spend much time actually doing the archival legwork necessary to arrive at the conclusion that treatment in the past was less effective than it is now.

However, a few researchers will cast a shadow on the handed-down success story. For example:

> Obsessive-compulsive disorder (OCD) continues to present a particular challenge to clinicians. As opposed to other anxiety disorders and, to some degree, to depression, the results of therapies, be they pharmacologic or psychological, are at best less than optimal. Indeed, when one reads articles reporting randomized controlled trials, patients are said to be responders when a 35% reduction of symptoms occurs (as if reducing rituals from 6 to 4 hours were clinically meaningful). Moreover, when one takes into account those who drop out of studies because of medication side effects or because of fear in the exposure-response prevention (ERP) studies—often in the 25% to 30% range—and add to those numbers the nonresponders, then we are looking at a 35% to 50% response in about 50% of patients. Additionally, few patients attain full remission—hardly satisfactory outcomes![55]

This pessimistic note is echoed by another researcher who writes, "Only one-half of OCD patients experience significant benefits from SSRIs. Further, when patients respond to treatment, the improvement is most often partial. Indeed, the OCD treatment-response criterion is generally an improvement of only 35% (and 25% in some cases) on the Yale-Brown Obsessive Compulsive Scale, whereas in depression a 50% amelioration is the norm."[56] It is important to recall that a 35 percent rate would be only a few points, if any, over placebo, and 25 percent would actually be worse than placebo.

A case in point can be made about the uptick success story concerning the placebo effect in OCD. It is generally held that if you give a group of people a placebo without their knowing that the pill contains no active ingredients, about a third of those people will report an improvement in their symptoms. So drug tests, when they say that 40 percent of the patients "improved," will actually be saying that only 7 percent really improved, since 33 percent or so would have improved simply because of the placebo effect. How then to account for a roundup article published in 2000 which noted that "in 1990, it was firmly asserted that there was a 'virtual absence' of placebo response in OCD." The data from early pharmacological trials of clomipramine that reported a low placebo response rate of about 5 to 10 percent were considered to confirm the rule, with some negligible exceptions. In this respect, OCD was held to be strikingly different from the anxiety and depressive disorders, where placebo response rates consistently fell between 30 and 50 percent. But in the ten years between 1990 and 2000, the figures for placebo effects mainly from SSRI trials began to increase, now ranging from 15 percent to the rather normal 30 percent, and even as high as 35.4 percent. With some studies showing the effectiveness rate of SSRIs at 38 percent, we may now be thinking of a mere 2.6 percent difference between placebo and drug. As the writers of the article conclude, "In the course of a few years, therefore, both available data and belief in its validity have changed dramatically from asserting 'virtual absence' of placebo response in OCD to the latest finding that every third OCD patient may be a placebo-responder."[57]

SELF-HELP BOOKS AND MEMOIRS

Paradoxes like these only add to a general confusion about the mechanisms, tests for, and results of research on OCD. Despite all these problems, as the OCD promotion continues, self-help books and media presentations simplify even further the quandaries and present the issue as rather obvious. The stream of information about the disease entity swirls through the media, self-help books, memoirs, and word of mouth so that a recognizable symptom pool develops. Individuals, family, and friends can "know" these symptoms, find them in a friend or relative, "understand" what needs to be done, and place the simplified and streamlined disease entity within a confident and knowing treatment regimen. First-person narratives in book form or on shows like *Oprah* provide compelling portals through which such information flows.

Take Emily Colas, whose book *Just Checking: Scenes from the Life of an Obsessive-Compulsive* is a very funny, sad, and highly readable book about OCD. Written in 1998 during the wild optimism about SSRIs, the following excerpt reads like a panacea for OCD:

> You can try really hard not to get better. Use all your strength and will. But when you're on the pill, you get better and there's not a whole lot you can do about it. It takes a little while to kick in, so there are about four or five

weeks when you're basically taking medication for the sheer benefit of the side effects. . . . But then it happens. Not dramatically. It comes on slowly, but you can tell. The thoughts and worries become less gripping.[58]

Cure no longer requires arduous psychotherapy or behavioral therapy. Instead there is just the automatic response to a drug trailing triumphantly behind a few pesky side effects. The individual testimony is only anecdotal evidence, but the force of the narrative form gives the attestation a special force.

And there's Marc Summers's confident lay assessment (aided by the helpful preposition "with," as in "with Eric Hollander, MD," as the cover byline proclaims): "Seventy-percent of OCD patients responded to treatment with Anafranil, which affects the serotonin system in the brain. This was a tremendous discovery. For the first time, doctors realized OCD was a treatable illness."[59] And about his experience on Luvox, he writes: "So, Dr. Hollander recommended I . . . try 75 milligrams daily. I started to notice a difference. Suddenly, I didn't have the need to straighten as much. It was the strangest feeling. . . . When Dr. Hollander upped my dosage to 100 milligrams, the effect was incredible. The desire to arrange and rearrange disappeared."[60] Again, the automatic relief from simply taking a pill is palpable. The very nature of self-help books, particularly first-person ones, is that they trace a heroic path from a low point of disease and disorder to a high point of triumph over despair. G. Thomas Couser has highlighted this trajectory in disability narratives.[61] So the glib successes I cited above glide over the actual difficulty of treating OCD, the low cure rate, and the lifetime nature of the disorder. Marc Summers, who gives us a version of the drug-success story, does later add that "very few people are fully 'cured' of OCD. I expect a continuous battle to keep my symptoms at bay for the rest of my life. It's day-to-day war, and most days I'm winning."[62] Summers uses the language of "relapse" to explain the contradiction between the idea of a successful endgame therapy and the idea of a never-ending war. Summers describes a relapse that he attributes to stress and discontinuation of medications, telling us that after going through an OCD episode, "I snapped out of my relapse." Note now that any medical intervention or drug effect is discarded. He simply "snaps" out. Summers continues: "I've had other relapses since then, and now I can predict when they'll happen. I'll be overloaded, spread too thin, trying to satisfy everybody."[63] This description contains a crucial contradiction.

If drug and behavioral therapy fix the broken brain, how do relapses occur? If Summers had symptoms after he went off medication, and then he "snapped" out of his relapse, how does that explain the idea of treatment and cure? If he goes back into OCD when he's stressed, then is stress the cause of OCD? A trigger? The whole thrust of the previous explanation is to promote the serotonin hypothesis and the broken-brain one. Now we're talking about stress and being "spread too thin"?

But messy relapses get in the way of the self-help narrative. So when self-help books get to tell this story, they usually flatten the bumps into the smooth narrative of cumulative knowledge, expertise, and success: "Spectacular improvement is the rule [for OCD]. . . . The great news for OCD sufferers is that obsessive-compulsive disorder is now recognized as a common, physical disease for which effective treatment is available."[64] Any doubts, complexities, and difficulties of the disorder disappear behind a glowingly edited history. The difficulties of treatment are brushed aside with an emphasis on responsiveness. But response to drugs or therapy can be represented by a mere few percentage points of improvement on scales always rated by a researcher or attested to by someone in a research protocol. Many studies will fail to say how much of a response we are considering, and fewer still are willing to acknowledge problems in their methods for assessment.

In a case described by Judith Rapoport, we can see embedded in the official triumphalist narrative this contradiction between the highlighted success story and the persistent failure story. In this case, she is discussing a patient named Charles, whom she put on Anafranil:

> Charles remained free of all symptoms for a year. And then they returned even though he was taking the medicine regularly. . . . Charles still isn't completely cured. In spite of the dramatic improvement with Anafranil, he can hide his ritual activity by performing in the evening when he is alone. . . . Charles had no response to Anafranil, and only modest improvement with behavior therapy. But he continues to fight these urges, and remains optimistic that help will come.[65]

A strange discontinuity appear here. Charles has had a "dramatic improvement with Anafranil," and yet he had "no response to Anafranil." Rapoport probably could have used a better editor, but the discontinuity isn't simply one of editorial consistency. Rather it reflects the built-in contradiction of the celebratory arc of the self-help book combined with the stubborn realities of OCD. Doctors want their patients to improve. Patients want to improve, but then a reality of the disorder sets in. It's a hard-to-treat condition that has ups and downs. In the 1970s OCD was described as an episodic disorder that had a low but consistent recovery rate and it remains this way now. Studies and research protocols can indeed find differences between people who take drugs or engage in behavioral therapy and those who don't. But the volume of hype about the success of these therapies is clearly turned up way too high.

INTERNET INTERVENTIONS

The Internet is rife with Web sites and links concerning OCD. Success, again, is the name of the game. Even reputable clinics are involved in the hype. Unlike peer review journals and even books, the Internet is a kind of Wild West for staking claims on the OCD mother lode. Since clinics and physicians can improve their business by making larger claims for success with OCD, optimism must rule in such unregulated settings. So despite pessimistic outlooks for OCD, physicians' Web sites will claim ridiculously high rates of success. For example, a web interview with John Calamari, PhD, associate professor and director of the Anxiety & OCD Treatment and Research Program at the Finch University of Health Sciences in North Chicago, yields this optimistic assessment: "Approximately 80% of individuals who start treatment achieve significant symptom reduction. It has been my clinical observation that those who don't benefit are unable or unwilling to stop ritualizing."[66] This statement was part of an interview by the OCD Foundation, and the format does not allow for footnotes, explanations of how Dr. Calamari arrived at his figures, and so on. But it is worth noting that the key phrase "significant symptom reduction" is ambiguous at best and subjective at worst. Further, the interesting move of removing those who don't benefit as people who are "unable or unwilling to stop ritualizing" is both tautological and dismissive. Is the 80 percent reduction in symptoms only among those who are willing and able? In that case, the 80 percent could hardly be a true 80 percent.

Another interview elicits the statement, "At the end of the intensive phase there is an average rate of 75 percent reduction in symptoms. After that, the patient continues treatment on a weekly basis dealing with his/her residual symptoms."[67] The confident statement is not accompanied by any documentation that would allow a check on its accuracy. It also contains the same wiggle phrase "reduction in symptoms." But further, the notion of "residual symptoms" begs the question of whether "symptom reduction" reduced the number of symptoms or the intensity. The 70–80 percent number is repeated in many other interviews, such as the statement, "Statistically, 70–80% of patients completing the treatment program achieve a clinically significant improvement in their OCD symptoms. Although we do not speak of patients as being cured, they complete the program with their OCD under control and they are armed with the tools that will help them to maintain their gains and, in many cases, to avoid major relapses."[68] But somehow the 70–80 percent cure rate fails to make it into the peer-reviewed journal articles. We can only assume that the anecdotal experience of these OCD clinics is not borne out by the harder numbers of research protocols.

It is understandable that researchers, practitioners, and patients all want to see improvement and cure. Like any other culture, the culture of OCD has its own narratives, myths, and ways of seeing the world. Interested parties will create explanations that interest them. Even controlled and scientific studies find it hard to eliminate bias. It isn't my purpose in this chapter to dash hopes and criticize the best work we currently have. I have simply wanted to show that we must be as scrupulous and suspicious of claims made in the name of science as we are about those made in the name of the arts or the humanities. If anything, I hope this chapter, and the book as well, demonstrates the virtues of biocultural criticism and discussion, so that we can consider things like brain scans and chemical analyses to be as subject to an informed discussion as we would consider *Moby-Dick* or the work of Van Gogh.

9

Conclusion: So What? So What? So What? So What? and Other Obsessive Thoughts

Every reader and every writer will have a moment when he or she pauses in the midst of a book and asks the fateful and perhaps devastating question—"So what?" If you ask that question enough times, you may even stop reading or writing—perhaps to the benefit of all. So if you've come along on this disquisition into obsession thus far, you may well now be asking that very question. If you are a medical practitioner or a person with OCD, you may especially be asking this question. After all, the author of this book is not a physician, not a researcher, not a clinician. What expertise could I possibly be offering to anyone who works in the trenches with patients or in the laboratory with expensive hi-tech machinery?

The argument I've been making in the book, explicitly and implicitly, is that you can't understand a disease like OCD without a thoroughgoing knowledge of the social, cultural, historical, anthropological, and political view of that entity. In effect, I'm arguing for what David Morris and I have been calling a "biocultural" approach. In our "Biocultures Manifesto" we make the point this way:

> Biology—serving at times as a metaphor for science—is as intrinsic to the embodied state of readers and of writers as history and culture are intrinsic to the professional bodies of knowledge known as science and biology. To think of science without including an historical and cultural analysis would

be like thinking of the literary text without the surrounding and embedding weave of discursive knowledges active or dormant at particular moments. It is similarly limited to think of literature—or to engage in debate concerning its properties or existence—without considering the network of meanings we might learn from a scientific perspective.[1]

Since we began separating science and the humanities in the nineteenth century, we have certainly had some major gains, but there are conceptual and methodological losses. Both science and the humanities are in need of each other, particularly in some complex arenas. What I've been trying to show is that in the area of certain kinds of psychiatric disorders, no single approach will yield as much information as a combined biocultural approach. The laboratory researchers will be limited by the *DSM* definition of the disease entity and will try to find places in the genes or the brain where anomalies show up given that definition. But that *DSM* definition itself, as we have seen, is mutable and determined by many social and cultural factors. The clinician will be limited by the definitional problem and the limited range of prescribed treatments, at this point mainly pharmaceutical and cognitive-behavioral. The patient will be limited to a strictly medical model of symptoms and diagnosis. The medical historian may also be limited by a lack of clinical and research experience. The point is that no one—therefore—can be an expert in OCD. Each person can only be an expert in OCD as envisioned by the parameters of his or her own field and profession. And that perspective, as I hope I have shown, will necessarily be limited.

But given what I've just said, it still could be expected that clinicians might respond with the "So what?" question.

As Wittgenstein once said, there are no commonsense answers to philosophical questions. I could therefore respond and say that any attempt to turn a historical and theoretical account of obsession into something utilitarian would be beside the point. I have in fact responded to questions from physicians by saying, "Your job is to work with patients, mine to work with ideas." It's equally true that at the end of the day, I have only pages to look at and not suffering people staring at me in my office.

Indeed, the recourse to suffering is the most consistent one that physicians use when they want to refute my work by producing their bona fides. Even those physicians most sympathetic to my project end up saying, "It's all well and good to think of OCD as having a history and thinking of it as a disease entity, but what do I do when confronted with a patient who is suffering?" The object of medicine is, after all, to relieve suffering.

And that is a valid point. But, although I'm not a physician and do not see patients, I have a counterexample to present. At a recent conference on the psychiatric consumer movement, after I'd presented a talk on obsession, a man came up to me and said, "I've had OCD my whole life." He proceeded to tell me about all the drugs he'd taken, the professionals he'd consulted. He obviously knew much about OCD and the full range of cures and treatments available. He told me that not much had helped, that he'd had cycles of intense OCD and times when it was less intense and more manageable. But then he said, "Your talk made me feel completely different about myself." I asked him to elaborate, and he said that knowing there was a history to his disorder, that there were famous people who had it, that it was a disease of rationality, was extremely important for his own sense of worth. In other words, he was telling me that having a new biocultural narrative about his illness, placing it in a social and historical context, was itself of therapeutic use.

Granted, this anecdote is only an anecdote. Yet it and the weight of the research of this book lead me to propose a biocultural experiment. Since science relies on hard data, a next step might be to test the hypothesis that giving doctors and patients a historical and social context into which they can place a disease entity might improve treatment rates, management, and outcomes for people with OCD. Such a proposal sounds strange or even impossible only because the climate of opinion in the medical world tends to minimize the effect of such kinds of knowledges in notions of cure.

One area where there has been success, though, has been in what has come to be called "narrative medicine" and particularly what Bradley Lewis has called "narrative psychiatry." Narrative has become a keyword in medical humanities and medical education. Rita Charon pioneered the field and many others, including Arthur Kleinman, David Morris, and G. Thomas Couser, have written about the value of narrative in medicine.[2] As Charon notes:

Many of us within medicine and within literary studies have realized the critical importance that writing—autobiography, memoir, pathography, fiction, personal essay—has developed within health care. Patients and their families are giving voice to their suffering, finding ways to write of illness and to articulate—and therefore comprehend—what they endure in sickness. The therapeutic potential of narrative medicine expands when we encourage patients to join us in writing their own medical charts, for patients are, or should be, the co-authors and curators of whatever records are kept about them. Health professionals, too, are writing reflective essays about their practice for medical journals or the trade press (Bolton). By *telling* of what we undergo in illness or in the care of the sick, we are coming to recognize the layered consequences of illness and to acknowledge the fear and hope and love exposed in sickness.[3]

The thrust of narrative medicine has been to give voice to the experience of being a patient, caregiver, family member, or doctor. The endeavor of engaging in narrative is itself seen as therapeutic for the patient. Moreover, Charon is currently involved in quantitative research aiming to show that physicians who engage in narrative through reading and writing actually are better practitioners than those who don't. It is this kind of research that could be fruitfully extended to the OCD question. Why not find out if there is a beneficial relationship between historical and cultural contextualizing and treatment outcomes, between understanding and improvement?

Felicia Aull and Bradley Lewis go a step further and introduce the idea that there is a social-cultural zone inhabited by patient and physician over which neither of them has control.[4] This space determines meanings and shapes relationships, and so Aull suggests a cultural studies approach as an addition to Charon's ideas of narrative medicine. Aull hopefully proposes, "If medical professionals are familiar with scholarship that underlies these movements, there is greater likelihood that they can work productively with such individuals or groups, and help to educate others."[5]

However, an area that has been largely overlooked by narrative medicine is the idea I am proposing, that the history of a disease itself constitutes a therapeutic narrative. We can think of disease biographies (as opposed to biographies by people with diseases) as fleshing out the social-cultural space that Aull and Lewis discuss. In other words, the cultural studies space, which includes the history of doctor-patient relations, could be usefully expanded to include the genesis of a disease in a culture. Not only am I talking about the history of disease; I am also trying to trace the borderlines between disease entities that have been mapped out in various times and places and other behaviors or bodily states that exist within the culture and are not called diseases. In the case of obsession, I've traced the pathological and the normative kinds of obsession, as well as the instantiations of obsession in valued visual and literary productions.

The effect of bringing in disease biographies (not only the biographies of people with diseases) will be in large part an educational effect. What is in essence a biocultural knowing of diseases can empower patients as well as physicians to rethink the way that disease is enforced and distributed through cultures and represented in popular and professional imaginations. As with my interlocutor who has learned that his obsessive behavior has a grand and admirable history, there may be therapeutic effects. Can we think of a changed society with a biocultural consciousness as one that has a new kind of control over disease? In this case, the disease isn't controlled through cure and eradication, although those goals are always worthy ones, but through a systematic rethinking of the way disease is structured and positioned in our society. If knowledge is power, then knowledge of disease amounts to a kind of power over that disease. Particularly in the cases of mental disorders, the way we think about the disease entity has a lot to do with how the "sufferer" regards his or her condition. This is even more so in the case of obsession since, according to Rachman, some aspect of OCD has to do with not being able to accept the notion that unacceptable ideas can obsess us.[6]

In a sense what I am describing might be seen as an attempt to decrease the gap between disease and illness. The former is the term most likely associated with a diagnosis, and the latter as the felt and lived experience of the person. That gap, detailed by Arthur Kleinman and David Morris, among others, has been used as a way into the patient's experience and narrative about his or her body. It was largely a defensive way of thinking, protecting the patient's body from being run over roughshod by a medical establishment. But we can also say that the distinction between disease and illness begins to collapse when we have elaborated more nuanced and detailed notion of how behaviors and states become diseases. That more complex approach would necessarily bring together the patient's experience with the clinician's expertise—would unpack the very nature of experience on both sides of the equation. Further, it would help the patient understand the nature of the clinician's expertise, and would allow the clinician to see the patient as a collaborator in the historical understanding of what it is that they are both doing.

In comparison with the rather crude set of diagnoses and cures that have evolved around obsession over the historical period we have looked at, a multifaceted approach that takes its impetus from such refined methodologies as are used in anthropology, cultural studies, literary and art criticism, philosophy, and history could be salutatory on many fronts. In any case, it would bring more narratives and perhaps better ones to the unexamined assumptions behind the current set of disorganized and somewhat desperate attempts to unify a shifting and elusive disease.

Bioethics tends to concern itself with the major principles of beneficence, autonomy, nonmalfeasance, informed consent, and justice. In these areas the crucial thing is that one should have access to a qualified physician who will act ethically by providing information accurately to the patient, obtaining informed consent for treatment and generally alleviating suffering while doing no harm. But in the scenario I've been describing, would it be possible for a physician to do all of the above in treating someone with OCD and still act unethically? The nodal points of interaction with the patient might all be filled with ethical concerns, but the seemingly neutral act of assigning a patient a diagnosis from the *DSM* may indeed, given our discussion, have its unethical aspects. As we have seen, the diagnosis of OCD does not come free and clear of a welter of concerns. These may not be the standard concerns of bioethics, but cumulatively they pose substantial areas of concern in the act of diagnosis.

I will grant that most psychiatrists and psychotherapists would have very little choice in diagnosing if they did not use the *DSM,* and this study should not be construed as a major critique of the *DSM.* Rather, my point is that providing a professionally sanctioned diagnosis is not a simple act, nor an unproblematic one. We can always see the error of our ways when we look back in psychiatric history to the charnel house of abandoned disease entities like hysteria or pseudo-neurotic schizophrenia. So while we don't normally consider it a bioethical issue when a practitioner assigns an approved and vetted diagnosis, I am suggesting that we might want to reconsider this truism. Just as we now recognize the inutility of many of those long-passed diagnostic categories, we need to consider the social, cultural, and historical biography of a disease as part of any bioethical assessment. To diagnose without understanding the ontology of that diagnosis is like starting a war without understanding the history of the affected region.

WASHING OUR HANDS OF IT

In the last days of writing this book, I gave a talk on obsession at a small Midwestern college. My talk was well received by the members of the humanities faculty and the students who were working on bioculturally related subjects. But an economist in the audience made a testy, or as she put it, "challenging," comment about how I had forgotten to talk about the pain suffered by people with OCD, and didn't I think that at the base it was the pain that made the disease real? I could tell right away that this wasn't a purely academic subject for her, and when she approached me at the lectern at the end of the session, she told me that her husband had suffered from OCD for many years. He had obsessive thoughts that he would kill someone, and she felt that medical intervention saved him from suicide.

I'd have to be a pretty unconcerned person not to recognize that there are many people "with" OCD who are suffering the worst imaginable pain, who are doing or thinking things they would really rather not. These folks are wasting inordinate amounts of time and even damaging their bodies and their intimate relationships in a driven and unstoppable quest whose goal eludes even themselves. It has not been my aim in this work to minimize that pain or to minimize the work done by those devoted practitioners who aim to alleviate the suffering.

Pain and suffering, however, cannot be the proof of anything other than pain and suffering. The intensity of one's pain doesn't change paradigms or treatments, just as a child's crying at night shouldn't alter the list of needs the child has even if the child doesn't cry. To emphasize pain and suffering is as much a rhetorical move as it is a legitimate complaint. And pain and suffering don't counter the claim that obsession is a wide-ranging social, cultural, historical, and, yes, medical phenomenon.

Individual sufferers of obsessions and compulsions are one instance in a long narrative about obsessions and compulsions. Their pain and suffering are part of the story, but the pain and suffering don't start, end, or summarize the story any more than do other elements in the story.

Let me illustrate my point by emphasizing a news story of the moment. Right now the press is heavily covering Methicillin-resistant Staphylococcus aureus (MRSA). For the past years we've seen pandemic panics around avian flu, West Nile virus, Ebola, Lyme disease, and even anthrax in postal envelopes. We hear about these pandemics through the media, and we are told to avoid them by precautionary measures. One current Web site lists these precautions in regard to MRSA:

- Wash your hands. Use soap and water or an alcohol-based hand sanitizer. Also, wash thoroughly. Experts suggest that you wash your hands for as long as it takes you to recite the alphabet.
- Cover cuts and scrapes with a clean bandage. This will help the wound heal. It will also prevent you from spreading bacteria to other people.
- Do not touch other people's wounds or bandages.
- Do not share personal items like towels or razors. If you use any shared gym equipment, wipe it down before and after you use it. Drying clothes, sheets, and towels in a dryer—rather than letting them air dry—helps kill bacteria.

Other sources recommend taking one's shoes off upon entering the house.

The point is that when we begin to follow these instructions and others we begin to be recognizably compulsive. Counting to fifteen or reciting the alphabet while washing one's hands could easily fit into an obsessive-compulsive spectrum. Avoiding towels used by anyone else at home could fit too. If you add to this all the precautions we are taking, based on scientific studies, including our exercise regimens, eating habits, vitamin and herbal supplementation, sanitary practices, sexual behaviors, drinking habits (whether consuming eight cups of water a day, filtering our water, buying spring water, or making sure we have our daily glass of red wine)—it may seem clear that we are living in a world of obsessional panic. We protect our computers against viruses, squirt sanitizer on our hands after riding the subway or shaking hands with someone who seems to be coming down with a cold, use latex to filter out the unwanted germs, wipe down the gym equipment with handy antibacterial wipes provided by the facility, and so on and so on.

Are we fooling ourselves pretending that it is we who are normal and that those who are pathological are the ones who do some or all of these practices at home in secret? How much of the pain and suffering of people "with" OCD is attributed to their feeling that they are weird or different or even possessed? And is it only these designated diseased ones who are suffering? My twenty-four-year old daughter recently had to get a "smartphone" for her job. She lamented how horrible it was to be on call all the time, how annoying it was to have to check her e-mail frequently during the day. Being connected all the time is painful. I check my e-mail continuously throughout the day. (I just checked it after writing that sentence!) We suffer from the manifold requirements of modern life that make us focus on one thing, or many single things. We pay the price for having careers that involve repetitive attention, repetitive motions, single-minded focus. We pay the price for living in a chemically, radio-actively, microwave-filled dangerous and germ-laden environment. It's a norm that we are becoming obsessively focused on public transmission of germs.

So perhaps we all have to wash our hands of this. Washing our hands of this involves, I would lobby, the understanding that a disease like OCD is a subcategory of what we all do. That, therefore, we want to narrativize illness so that individuals "with" the disease can think of themselves as sharing it, not "having" it. They may have dipped into the stream a little too deeply, but we're all wading through this difficult current.

In psychoanalysis there is a term "isolation of affect." This is when emotional conflict is resolved with a defense mechanism that separates ideas from the feelings that accompany them. We can say that in some way society has perfected a collective defense mechanism called "isolation of illness." This mental quarantine walls off the diseased person from the rest of the population. It becomes very important to make strong and durable boundaries between diseases and between diseased populations. In the realm of cognitive and affective disorders, this collective quarantine can be performed to eliminate continua. Practitioners will say that there is no connection at all between the obsessive person and the obsessive society. I would say that this constitutes "isolation of illness." The patient's experience of his or her own internal state is separated out from the experience of the collectivity. It is given a diagnostic name, made into a disease, and the bond between patient and disease is reinforced. The patient becomes his or her disease. One moves from a person who is be-having as we all do, but perhaps more so, to a person who "has" OCD. The quarantine continues through the idea that family and friends will then treat the person as his or her disease, and the practitioner will treat the person as a disease to be cured. In any case, the isolation effort is agreed on all around, especially by the patient.

My point throughout this book is to question that isolation, to wonder about the durability and even legitimacy of the walls, to add to the richness of the disease phenomena by extending it from its quarantine to the society at large and moving it back and forth through the corridors of history. I hope to have made the point that a disease, like a person or a location, with a history is more understandable than a disease without one. If this book has accomplished anything, it has been as another chapter in the ongoing history of obsessions written by people who are obsessed with obsession. It won't be the last, since obsession, like guilt, is the gift that keeps giving.

Acknowledgments

Grateful thanks to the John Simon Guggenheim foundation for a fellowship to complete this work. Also thanks to the Department of English and the College of Liberal Arts at the University of Illinois at Chicago for their support of my research.

I am thus indebted for discussions, interventions, questions, and support to my colleagues at the University of Illinois at Chicago—Gerald Graff, Cathy Birkenstein, Walter Benn Michaels, Jennifer Ashton, Joseph Tabbi, Jenny Briar, John D'Emilio, Brenda Russell, Chris Comer, David Mitchell, Sharon Snyder, Carol Gill. Friends, colleagues, and interlocutors from outside Chicago include Bradley Lewis, Phil Alcabes, Jonathan Metzl, David Morris, Jennifer Fleisner, Nicole Anderson, Joseph Pugliesi, Catherine Mills, Rayna Rapp, Faye Ginsburg, Troy Duster, Emily Martin, Nikolas Rose, Marquard Smith, Joanne Morra, Berenice Hausman, Rebecca Garden, Richard Barney, Robert Markley, Nicholas Mirzoeff, Carol Nealy, Lynne Enterline, Barbara Katz-Nelson, Jonathan Lamb, Bridget Orr, Bruce Robbins, Jackie Orr, Stanley Fish, Jane Tompkins, Sally Weintrobe, Lez Weintrobe, Ralph Savarese, Jill Gage, Roberto De Romanis, Rosamaria Loretelli, and Brent Harold. For help with the working details of this book, thanks to my research assistants Alice Haisman and Aimee Wodda. And as always deep appreciation to my family members, Bella

Mirabella, Carlo Mirabella-Davis, and Francesca Mirabella, who keep the conversation going at all hours of the day.

Major thanks to the University of Chicago Press's able staff, particularly to Alan Thomas, who supported this project before it was even written. His continuing advice and editorial suggestions helped to make this a much more readable and elegant book. Thanks also to Carol Fisher Saller, whose editorial help smoothed out the rough edges and did so with humor and a light touch. Randy Petilos worked very hard to get my erratic notion of permissions in line with current practice; Isaac Tobin's brilliant cover design surprised and delighted me; and Stephanie Hlywak's enthusiasm and savvy helped to promote this book beyond the usual academic barriers.

Special thanks to Eric Zinner of New York University Press, who also supported this project in its early days, and whose suggestions, given over a few very pleasant dinners, immeasurably helped to improve the book. His grace and generosity throughout the process were as valuable as his advice.

Notes

INTRODUCTION

1 Pilar Viladas, "Obsession," *New York Times Magazine* (October 13, 2002), 65.

2 Rosemary Sullivan, *Labyrinth of Desire: Women, Passion, and Romantic Obsession* (Toronto: Harper*Flamingo,* 2001), 2.

3 http://www.gallup-robinson.com/essay65.html.

4 "The Culture of Mania," in *Subjectivity and Experience Transformed,* ed. Joao Biehl, Byron Good, and Arthur Kleinman (Cambridge: Harvard, 2005).

5 Ian Hacking, *Rewriting the Soul: Multiple Personality and the Science of Memory* (Princeton: Princeton University Press, 1995), pp. 8–20; and *Mad Travelers: Reflections on the Reality of Transient Mental Illnesses* (Charlottesville: University of Virginia, 1998), pp. 1–2; 51–102. Charles E. Rosenberg, "The Tyranny of Diagnosis: Specific Entities and Individual Experience," *Milbank Quarterly* 80:2 (2002), 237–60.

6 Rosenberg, 241.

7 http://www.psyweb.com/Mdisord/AnxietyDis/ocd1.html.

8 http://www.psyweb.com/Mdisord/ocpd.html.

9 The further revision incorporated into the *DSM-V* may in fact eliminate obsessive-compulsive personality as a diagnostic category.

10 Stanley J. Rachman and Ray J. Hodgson, *Obsessions and Compulsions* (Englewood, NJ: Prentice-Hall, 1980), 10.

11 Stanley J. Rachman, *The Treatment of Obsessions* (Oxford: Oxford University Press, 2003), 5.

12   Steven A. Rasmussen and Jane L. Eisen, "The Epidemiology and Clinical Features of Obsessive-Compulsive Disorder," in Michael Jenike, Lee Baer, William Minicheillo, *Obsessive-Compulsive Disorders: Practical Management* (New York: Mosby, 1998), 25.

13   Rachman and Hodgson, 3.

14   For more on the *DSM* in this regard see Geoffrey C. Bowker, *Sorting Things Out* (Cambridge, MA: MIT Press).

15   Lennard J. Davis, *Enforcing Normalcy: Disability, Deafness, and the Body* (London: Verso, 1995).

16   Rachman and Hodgson, 12.

17   Rachman and Hodgson, 13.

18   Susan Sontag, *Aids and Its Metaphors* (New York: Random House, 1979).

19   Lennard Davis and David Morris, "Biocultures Manifesto," *NLH* 38 (Fall 2007), 411–18.

20   Rachmand and Hodgson, 18.

21   See William Van Ornum, *A Thousand Frightening Fantasies: Understanding and Healing Scrupulosity and Obsessive Compulsive Disorder* (New York: Crossroads, 1997).

22   Rachman and Hodgson, 94.

23   There is a further critique to make of the prejudice toward the use of numbers in a statistical mode. And we will want to keep alert to the rise of statistics as a phenomenon of the very same modernity we are ourselves regarding. In this context, we should recall that the founding of the Statistical Society in London began with the assemblage of a group of men, all of whom were eugenicists, who inaugurated a mode of thinking that has become very common now, but which carried with it an entire set of presuppositions about human life and its relation to numbers.

24   Rachman and Hodgson, 21.

25   Rachman, 15.

26   I should note that from a psychoanalytic perspective, the content of the obsession is relatively irrelevant. The principal is that obsessional neurosis is characterized by a divorce of the symptom from the cause, a defense in which the activity provided by obsession is a diversion or a distraction from the motivating cause. In this line of thinking the obsessional activity does not particularly matter and is chosen for its arbitrary distance from the originating cause of unwanted sexual or aggressive impulses. However, most practitioners now disregard a psychoanalytic explanation of OCD.

27   Rachman and Hodgson, 254.

28   John E. Grant, Anthony Pinto, Matthew Gunnip, et al., "Sexual obsessions and clinical correlates in adults with obsessive-compulsive disorder," *Comprehensive Psychiatry* 47:5 (September–October 2006), 325–29.

29   Naomi Finberg, Donatella Marazziti, Dan J. Stein, eds., *Obsessive Compulsive Disorder: A Practical Guide* (London: Dunitz, 2001), 7.

30   There is an institutional history to the distinction between personality type and disorder. Freud noted the distinction between the anal type of personality and the obsessive neurotic. Ernest Jones and Karl Abraham reiterated the distinction. In the 1960s Joseph Sandler developed tests to distinguish between the personality type (which he called Type A) and the disorder (which he called Type B). The *DSM-IV TR* followed that distinction, although there is an indication that the *DSM-V* will abandon the personality type as a pathological entity. Eric Hollander and others have reversed the trend of firewalling distinctions between these types by introducing the notion of an OCD continuum.

31   Rachman and Hodgson, 58.

32   Dana J. H. Niehaus and Dan J. Stein, "Obsessive-Compulsive Disorder: Diagnosis and Assessment" in Eric Hollander, ed., *Obsessive-Compulsive Disorder: Diagnosis, Etiology, Treatment* (London: Informa, 1997), 4.

33   Rachman and Hodgson, 98.

34   Rachman and Hodgson, 99.

35   See David Morris, *Illness and Culture in the Postmodern Age* (Berkeley: University of California Press, 2000).

36   Indeed, the more we learn about genomics, the more we realize that while humans are very similar, significant individual differences in our DNA can make us react quite differently to the same environment.

37   Obviously, even with these physical diseases, there is a large range of variation which observers have smoothed out in order to create agreed-upon diagnostic categories.

38   See Bradley Lewis, *Moving Beyond Prozac, DSM, and the New Psychiatry: The Birth of Postpsychiatry* (Ann Arbor: University of Michigan Press, 2006).

39   Sylvere Lotringer, ed., *Foucault Live: Collected Interviews, 1961–1984* (New York: Semiotexte, 1996), 197.

40   Juliet Mitchell, *Mad Men and Medusas: Reclaiming Hysteria* (New York: Basic Books, 2000), 13.

41   See Georges Canguilhem, *On the Normal and the Pathological,* trans. R. Fawcett (New York: Zone Books, 1991).

42   See for example Nikolas Rose, "Neurochemical Selves," *Society* (November/December 2003), 46–59.

43   D. S. Weisberg, F. C. Keil, J. Goodstein, and J. Grey, "The Seductive Allure of Neuroscience Explanations," *Journal of Cognitive Neuroscience* (forthcoming); paper available at http://pantheon.yale.edu/-dis73/Assets/Weisberg-neuro%20explanations.pdf.

44   Rosenberg, 248.

45　Edith Rüdin, "Ein Beitrag zur Frage der Zwangskrankheit insbesondere ihrer hereditären Beziehungen," *Archiv für Psychiatrie und Zeitschrift Neurologie* 191 (1953), 14–54; cited in Paul Adams, *Obsessive Children* (New York: Penguin, 1973), 209. Actually, although this is impossible to prove, many studies end up with this tri-part conclusion, which is perhaps a function of bell-curve results in poorly planned protocols.

46　See for instance L. R. Baxter, J. M. Schwartz, K. S. Bergman, M. P. Szubba, B. H. Guze, J. C. Mazziotta, et al., "Caudate Glucose Metabolic Rate Changes with Both Drug and Behavior Therapy for Obsessive-Compulsive Disorder," *Archives of General Psychiatry* 49 (1992), 681–89; or J. Schwartz, P. Stoesse, L. Baxter, K. Martin, and M. Phelps, "Systematic Changes in Cerebral Glucose Metabolic Rate after Successful Behavior Modification Treatment of OCD," *Archives of General Psychiatry* 53 (1996), 109–13.

47　Benedict Carey, "For Psychotherapy's Claims, Skeptics Demand Proof," *New York Times,* August 10, 2004, F1.

CHAPTER ONE

1　Christian Renous, "Possession and Obsession in the XVIIth Century: Diagnosis and Treatment," *Healing, Magic, and Belief in Europe: 15th–20th Centuries New Perspectives* (Zeist, Netherlands: Conference Centre Woudschoten, 1994), 208.

2　While the devil explanation now seems archaic, at least one psychiatrist notes, "It must be said at the outset that attributing the cause of obsessions to the intrusions of the Devil is more immediately understandable than ascribing them to the vagaries of infant bowel training." Rachman and Hodgson, 22.

3　Michel Foucault objects to the "myth" of the derivation of madness from witchcraft and demonology (Lotringer, 196.) In the case of obsession, he appears to be incorrect, since the very word is linked to the discourse surrounding the devil.

4　According to a 1398 reference in the *OED.*

5　Richard Hunter and Ida Macalpine, *Three Hundred Years of Psychiatry,* 1535–1860 (Oxford: Oxford University Press, 1963; reprinted 1964), 357.

6　All information on this event comes from "Country News," *Gentleman's Magazine* 57:1 (1787), 268.

7　Electrical devices based on friction were commonly used in England at fairs and public events by the mid-eighteenth century. Benjamin Franklin had suggested using electricity on mad people.

8　John Friend, "De spasmi rarioris historia," *Philosophical Transactions* (1701) cited in Hunter and Macalpine, *Three Hundred Years of Psychiatry,* 506.

9   Gabriel Tarde, "Foules et sectes au point de vue criminal," *Revue des deux mondes* 120 (November 15, 1893), 349–87, trans. Kathleen Marien, cited in Athena Vrettos, *Somatic Fictions: Imagining Illness in Victorian Culture* (Stanford: Stanford University Press, 1995), 81.

10 Robert Whytt, *Works* (Edinburgh: J. Balfour, 1768), 487.

11 Anna Vila, "Beyond Sympathy: Vapours, Melancholia, and the Pathologies of Sensibility in Tissot and Rousseau," *Yale French Studies* (1997), 89.

12 Thomas Willis, *An Essay on the Pathology of the Brain and Nervous Stock* (London: J. B. for T. Dring, 1681).

13 Klaus Doerner, *Madmen and the Bourgeoisie: A Social History of Insanity and Psychiatry,* trans. Joachim Neugroschel and Jean Steinberg (Oxford: Blackwell, 1981), 25.

14 Hysteria has had a resurgence recently as a legitimate rather than fanciful illness. Brain scans indicate a somatic origin for hysteria. See, for example, Omar Ghaffar, W. Richard Staines, and Anthony Feinstein, "Unexplained Neurologic Symptoms: An fMRI Study of Sensory Conversion Disorder," *Neurology* 67 (2006), 2036–38.

As with all aspects of madness, it is wise to be proactive so as to preempt the ideological reflex one might call "normalization" of mental states. That is, when we read that "possession" was the operative term for madness in Shakespeare's time, we will immediately defend ourselves by feeling a kind of automatic superiority to a culture that has the silly or primitive idea of possession or witchcraft. We must, throughout this enterprise, instead interrogate the validity of our own concepts rather than employ a smug superiority to the categories of the past or the categories of other cultures. Just as religion is seen as what we believe to be true and myth what the Greeks and other ancient cultures falsely believed, we might use this foray as an exercise in contemplating the categorization of mental and emotional states. Juliet Mitchell helps us do that by pointing out that hysteria, for example, might indeed be a universal category rather than a time-bound and hidebound idea. She speaks of the Taita people on the coast of Kenya who have an illness they call *saka,* which they describe as an illness of "wanting and wanting." Western observers have called the disease "Possession 'Hysteria.'" Mitchell's point is that "hysteria is a universal phenomenon, a possible response to particular human conditions that can arise at any time or anywhere" (Mitchell, 13). Ian Hacking's *Mad Travellers,* too, reminds us that the categories of mental illness are "transient," with each new formulated disease reflecting more our own way of categorizing and thinking than any specific organic or mental configuration. Thus, though we might not talk about demonic possession, we do have a language to discuss the way that outside forces take over and affect the mind. We may discuss the influence of media violence on high-school shooters or we may discuss how child abuse creates adult abusers. We may not accept hysteria or the vapors, but we have plenty of diseases that affect our emotional states with depression, lethargy, nervousness, anomie, addictions, and so on. We somehow feel that if we can find a drug that affects the emotional state described by a known disease entity, say depression, that we have identified the disease. But we forget that bromides, bloodletting, cupping, herbal remedies, rest cures, and other past treatments were quite effective, according to physicians and patients, in alleviating symptoms. The history of mental illness and its treatment is not simply a failure in the past and a success in the present.

15   The contemporary meaning of "hypochondria"—concern over imagined diseases—did not occur until later.

16   George Cheyne, *The English Malady* (London: Wisk, Ewing, and Smith, 1733),179–80.

17   Thomas Arnold, *Observations on the Nature, Kinds, Causes, and Prevention of Insanity, Lunacy, or Madness* (London, G. Robinson, 1882), 1:29.

18   Arnold, 1:30.

19   For a view of hysteria as a particularly female disease of the nineteenth and twentieth centuries see the influential work by Elaine Showalter, *The Female Malady: Women, Madness, and English Culture, 1830–1980* (New York: Pantheon, 1985) as well as Georges Didi-Huberman, *Invention of Hysteria: Charcot and the Photographic Iconography of Salpêtrière*, trans. Alisa Hartz (Cambridge, MA: MIT Press, 2003). For a more contemporary view of hysteria, see Mitchell.

20   Cheyne to Richardson, July 1742, in *The Letters of Doctor George Cheyne to Samuel Richardson (1733–1743)*, ed. Charles F. Mullett (New York: Columbia University Press, 1943), 104; also cited in Anita Guerrini, *Obesity and Depression in the Enlightenment: The Life and times of George Cheyne* (Norman: University of Oklahoma Press, 2000), 6.

21   Cheyne, *The English Malady*, i–ii; cited in Andrew Scull, *The Most Solitary of Afflictions: Madness and Society in Britain 1700–1900* (New Haven: Yale University Press, 1993), 179. This number obtains pretty consistently through the variety of broadly applied mental illnesses named variously hysteria, neurasthenia, neurosis, anxiety, depression, and so on.

22   Henry Mackenzie, *The Man of Feeling* (1771; reprinted New York: Norton, 1958), 19.

23   William Harvey, "Anatomical Exercises on the Generation of Animals . . ." (1651); reprinted in *The Works of William Harvey, M.D.*, ed. and trans. Robert Willis (London, 1847), 542.

24   Cheyne, *The English Malady*, i–ii.

25   Cheyne, *The English Malady*, 262.

26 George Cheyne, *An Essay of Health and Long Life* (London: George Strahan, 1724), 171, 158; cited in Guerrini, 123.

27 David Hume to [George Cheyne?], ca. March 1734, in David Hume, *The Letters of David Hume,* ed. J. Y. T. Greig (Oxford: Clarendon Press, 1932), 1:15; cited in Guerrini, 123.

28 Cheyne, *English Malady,* 105; cited in Guerrini, 147.

29 Scull, 180.

30 H. C. Erik Midelfort, "Madness and the Problems of Psychological History in the Sixteenth Century," *Sixteenth Century Journal* 12:1 (Spring 1981), 8; Doerner, 40.

31 Bartholomaeus Anglicus, *De proprietatibus rerum* (1535), in Hunter and Macalpine, 1.

32 Ludwig Lavater, *Of Ghostes and Spirites Walking by Nyght* (London: Watkins, 1572), cited in Hunter and Macalpine, 17.

33 Philip Barrough, *The Method of Physicke* (London: Vautrollier, 1583), in Hunter and Macalpine, 27–28.

34 Reginald Scot, *The Discovery of Witchcraft* (London: Brome, 1584), in Hunter and Macalpine, 33.

35 In Hunter and Macalpine, 33.

36 Richard Baxter, *The Signs and Causes of Melancholy: With Directions Suited to the Case of Those Who Are Afflicted with It,* in Allan Ingram, *Patterns of Madness in the Eighteenth Century: A Reader* (Liverpool: Liverpool University Press, 1988), 43.

37 Bernard Mandeville, *A Treatise of the Hypochondriack and Hysterick Diseases,* in Ingram, 51.

38 Lavater; cited in Hunter and Macalpine, 17.

39 Arnold, 1:10.

40 Arnold, 1:9.

41 Immanuel Kant, *Anthropology from a Pragmatic Point of View,* trans. Mary J. Gregor (The Hague, Netherlands: Martinus Nijhoff, 1982), 83–84.

42 Ann Bristow, *The Maniac, a Tale; or, a View of Bethlem Hospital* (London: J. Hatchard, 1810).

43 J.-J. Belloc, *Cours de medicine légale, théorique et pratique* (Paris: Méquignon, 1819), 255–56 (originally published in 1800).

44 Urbain Coste, review of *Dictionnaire abrégé des sciences médicales,* in *Journal Universel des Sciences Médicales* 43 (1826), 53.

45 Hunter and Macalpine, 640.

46 Scull, 185.

47 Thomas Mayo, *Remarks on Insanity: Founded on the Practice of John Mayo, MD* (London: Underwood, 1817), in Scull, 207.

48 Guerrini, 98.

49   Scull, 179.

50   John Conolly, *An Inquiry Concerning the Indications of Insanity, With Sugges-tions for the Better Protection and Care of the Insane* (London: Taylor, 1830), 7; cited in Scull, 209.

51   Francis Willis, *A Treatise on Mental Derangement* (London: Longman, Hurst, Rees, Orme, and Brown, 1823; reprinted 1843), 2; cited in Scull, 207.

52   Richard Blackmore, *A Treatise of the Spleen and Vapours: Or, Hypochondriacal and Hysterical Affections* (London: Pemberton, 1725), 17.

53   James Boswell, *The Life of Samuel Johnson* (Boston: Charles E. Lauriat Co., 1925), 1:24.

54   William Battie, *A Treatise on Madness* (London: 1758), 7.

55   Alexander Anderson, *An Inaugural Dissertation on Chronic Mania* (New York: T. and Swords, 1796), 10.

56   John Locke, *An Essay concerning Human Understanding* (London: William Tegg, 1849), 94.

57   Battie, 7.

58   Basil Clarke points out in his *Mental Disorder in Earlier Britain* (Cardiff: University of Wales Press, 1975) that the number of mentally ill in early England was quite low.

59   All cited in Guerrini, 106.

60   A recent study of the American Psychological Association notes that money is the number one source of stress for 73 percent of Americans.

61   Anderson, 6.

62   Anderson, 6.

63   S. A. Tissot, *An Essay on Diseases Incidental to Literary and Sedentary Persons with Proper Rules for Preventing Their Fatal Consequences* (London: Edward and Charles Dilly, 1768), 39.

64   Arnold, 1:106, 108.

65   Anderson, 6.

66   G. S. Rousseau, "Science and the Discovery of the Imagination in Enlightened England," *Eighteenth-Century Studies* 3:1, Special Issue: *The Eighteenth-Century Imagination* (Autumn 1969), 123.

67   Hunter and Macalpine, 502.

68   Joel Peter Eigen, "Eighteenth-Century Insanity Defenses," in *The Anatomy of Madness: Essays in the History of Psychiatry,* ed. W. F. Bynum, Roy Porter, and Michael Shepherd (London: Tavistock, 1985), 2:36.

69   Eigen, 36.

70   Nigel Walker, *Crime and Insanity in England* (Edinburgh: Edinburgh University Press, 1968), 1:56.

71   Eigen, 37.

72   Thomas Erskine, "Speech for the Defence" in *A Complete Collection of State Trials,* ed. T. B. Howell (London: Longman, 1820), 27:1309–23.

73 Eigen, 42.

74 Mullett, 104.

75 Raymond Stephanson, "Richardson's 'Nerves': The Physiology of Sensibility in *Clarissa*," *Journal of the History of Ideas* 49:2 (April–June 1988), 284.

76 Thomas Bridges, *The Adventure of a Bank-Note,* 54; cited in Mackenzie, vi.

77 William Stukely, *Of the Spleen* (London, 1725), 25.

78 Christopher Hamlin, "Chemistry, Medicine, and the Legitimization of English Spas, 1740–1840," in *The Medical History of Waters and Spas,* ed. Roy Porter (London: Welcome Institute, 1990), 68–69.

79 Audrey Heywood, "A Trial of the Bath Waters: The Treatment of Lead Poisoning," in Porter, 89.

80 Arnold, 1:26.

81 Trotter, 29.

82 James Makittrick Adair, *Medical Cautions for the Consideration of Invalids, More Especially of Those Who Resort to Bath* (Bath: Dodsley & Dilly, 1786), cited in Hunter and Macalpine, 489.

83 William Cullen, *First lines in the Practice of Physic* (Edinburgh: C. Elliot, 1784), 3.1033.

84 Cheyne, *The English Malady,* 14; cited in Guerrini, 132.

85 Mackenzie, 19.

86 Trotter, 89.

87 Simon During, "The Strange Case of Monomania: Patriarchy in Literature, Murder in *Middlemarch,* Drowning in *Daniel Deronda,*" *Representations* 23 (Summer 1988), 91.

88 For much more on monomania, although with a distinctly Freudian perspective, see Marina Van Zuylen, *Monomania: The Flight from Everyday Life in Literature and Art* (Ithaca: Cornell University Press, 2005).

89 William Godwin, *Caleb Williams* (London: Penguin, 1988), 109.

90 The first official detective to appear in fiction is Inspector Bucket of the Bow Street Runners in *Bleak House* (1854) some sixty years after Godwin's work. Poe's Dupin, of the "Purloined Letter" (1845) and "The Murders of the Rue Morgue" (1841) appeared ten years earlier, although he is not an official detective but rather, like Sherlock Holmes, who first appeared in *Study in Scarlet* (1887), an inspired amateur. Dupin's obsession with details and rationality, a kind of hyperattentiveness to detail, fits into the full flowering of an analytic fascination with a particular solution to an event. Wilkie Collins's *The Moonstone* (1868) has a Sergeant Cuff, but the details of the story unfold in multiple narratives, placing the reader in the role of detective.

91 Godwin, 132.

92 Barbara Benedict, *Curiosity: A Cultural History of Early Modern Inquiry* (Chicago: University of Chicago Press, 2001), 237.

93   Godwin, 129.

94   See Helen Deutsch, *Loving Dr. Johnson* (Chicago: University of Chicago Press, 2005); and my book *Bending Over Backwards: Disability, Dismodernism, and Other Difficult Positions* (New York: New York University Press, 2002), 47–61.

95   Boswell, 1:24.

96   Thomas Babington Macaulay, *Life of Samuel Johnson* (Boston: Ginn and Company, 1904), 4.

97   Trotter, xvii.

98   Cheyne to Richardson, 2 May 1742, in Mullett, 104; also cited in Guerrini, 163.

99   Andrew Harper, *Treatise on the Real Cause and Cure of Insanity* (London: C. Stalker, 1789), 33.

100   Erasmus Darwin, *Zoonomia; or, The Laws of Organic Life* (London: Johnson, 1796), 350–53.

101   Arnold, 1:110.

102   Arnold, 2:318ff.

103   Alexander Crichton, *An Inquiry into the Nature and Origin of Mental Derangement* (London: T. Cadell, Junior, and W. Davies, 1798).

104   Tissot, 24.

105   Samuel Johnson, *Rasselas: Prince of Abyssinia* (Chicago: McClurg & Co., 1889), 172.

106   Johnson, 173.

107   Laurence Sterne, *The Life and Opinions of Tristram Shandy* (Harmondsworth: Penguin, 1967), 113.

108   Johann Wolfgang von Goethe, *The Sorrows of Young Werther,* trans. Catherine Hutter (New York: Signet, 1962), 108.

109   While Benedict sees curiosity at the end of the eighteenth century as a form of resistance to "the cultural march toward systematization, classification, and the regulation of morality and social behavior" (202), it is also possible to see curiosity as the leading edge of a social construction that is a symptom of systematization rather than a resistance to it.

110   *The Rambler* 4:186 (no. 103, Tuesday, 12 March 1750).

111   "Le grammairien et le causeur," *Journal de la langue français,* 3:2 (1839), 522 cited in Goldstein, 153.

112   Tissot, 43.

113   Sir Henry Holland, "On Dreaming, Insanity, Intoxication, etc.," in *Medical Notes and Reflections* (London: Longman, 1839), 240.

114   Michael J. Clarke, "'Morbid Introspection,' Unsoundness of Mind, and British Psychological Medicine, c.1830–1900," in Bynum, Porter, and Shepherd, 3:72.

CHAPTER TWO

1 "Monomania," *Journal de Médecine et de Chirugie Pratiques* (March 1856), translated and reprinted in *American Journal of Insanity* 13:1 (July 1856), 51.

2 "Monomania," 52.

3 During, 86. Quotation from Étienne Esquirol, *Mental Maladies: A Treatise on Insanity,* trans. E. K. Hunt (Philadelphia, 1845), 320.

4 Marcel Gauchet and Gladys Swain, *Madness and Democracy: The Modern Psychiatric Universe,* trans. Catherine Porter (Princeton: Princeton University Press, 1999), 40; originally published in French as *La pratique de l'esprit humain* (Paris: Gallimard, 1980).

5 Scull, 334–74.

6 Jan Goldstein, *Console and Classify: The French Psychiatric Profession in the Nineteenth Century* (New York: Cambridge University Press, 1987), 154.

7 Goldstein, 153.

8 Esquirol, 320.

9 Esquirol, 320.

10 Conolly, 292–93; cited in Scull, 346.

11 Cited in Goldstein, 158.

12 Goldstein, 158.

13 Esquirol, 36.

14 C. P. Collard de Martigny, "Examen médico-légal de l'opinion émise par divers medicines sur la monomanie homicide," *Questions de jurisprudence médico-légale* (Paris: Auger-Méquignon, 1828), 15; cited in Goldstein, 177.

15 Anon., "Insanity—My Own Case," *American Journal of Insanity* 13:1 (1956–57), 25.

16 Charles Dickens, *American Notes* (New York: Pollard and Moss, 1884), 240.

17 Mackenzie, 19.

18 Mary Shelley, *Frankenstein* (Oxford: Oxford University Press, 1969; reprinted 1990), 16.

19 For example, "I seemed to have lost all soul or sensation but for this one pursuit" (54), and "I was thus engaged, heart and soul, in one pursuit" (55).

20 Werner Meunsterberger, *Collecting: An Unruly Passion* (Princeton: Princeton University Press, 1994), 101ff.

21 Honoré de Balzac, *Old Goriot,* trans. Marion Ayton Crawford (Harmondsworth: Penguin, 1951; reprinted 1981), 71.

22 Esquirol, 39.

23 Esquirol, 39.

24 Philippe Pinel and Isidore Bricheteau, "Névrose," *Dictionnaire des sciences médicales* (Paris: Panckoucke, 1819), 571; cited in George F. Drinka, *The*

Birth of Neurosis: Myth, Malady, and the Victorians (New York: Simon and Schuster, 1984), 42.

25 Esquirol, 336.

26 Tissot, 41.

27 Tissot 108.

CHAPTER THREE

1 For study of schizophrenia and its relation to the modern era see Louis A. Sass, *Madness and Modernism: Insanity in the Light of Modern Art, Literature, and Thought* (New York: Basic Books, 1992).

2 Gauchet and Swain, 37.

3 Peacock, 39.

4 Sarah Hoare, *Poems on Conchology and Botany* (London: Simpkin and Marshall, 1831), 61.

5 In fact, the gold standard for experimentation with drugs—the double-blind, randomized study—was not put into effect until well into the 1960s, and is still more rarely done than might be suspected.

6 G. E. Berrios, "Obsessional disorders during the nineteenth century: terminological and classificatory issues," in *The Anatomy of Madness: Essays in the History of Psychiatry,* vol. 1, ed. W. F. Bynum, Roy Porter, and Michael Shepherd (London: Tavistock Publications, 1988), 166.

7 Bernard Howard, "A Luke Howard Miscellany: Compiled by His Great Grandson" (London: typescript, 1959), 138–39; in Richard Hamblyn, *The Invention of Clouds: How an Amateur Meteorologist Forged the Language of the Skies* (New York: Picador, 2001), 249.

8 Howard, 138–39; in Hamblyn, 249.

9 Francis Galton, *Memories of My Life* (London: Methuen, 1908), unnumbered preface.

10 Galton, 3.

11 Francis Galton, *The Art of Travel* (London: John Murray, 1872; reprinted London: Phoenix Press, 2000), xii.

12 That neurasthenia continued to be regarded as a serious category is illustrated by a short review that the young Freud wrote in 1887 in which he mentions that neurasthenia "may comfortably be described as the commonest of all the diseases in our society." Sigmund Freud, *Standard Edition of the Complete Psychological Works of Sigmund Freud,* trans. James Strachey, with Anna Freud (London: Hogarth Press, 1966) (hereafter referred to as *SE*) 1:35.

13 Galton, *Memories,* 154.

14 One wonders if Galton's experiments in suffocation were actually the commonly reported kind that adolescent boys engage in while masturbat-

ing. Obviously he could not report this type of activity in his memoir, but such practices would fit into his obsessive behaviors.

15   Galton, *Memories,* 185–86.

16   D. W. Forrest, *Francis Galton: The Life and Work of a Victorian Genius* (New York, Taplinger, 1974), 45; citing F. Galton, *Tropical South Africa* (London, 1853), 115.

17   Mrs. Mathews, *Memoirs of Charles Mathews, Comedian* (London: Richard Bently, 1839), 4:137; cited in Bernth Lindfors, "Ethnological Show Business: Footlighting the Dark Continent," in *Freakery: Cultural Spectacles of the Extraordinary Body,* ed. Rosemarie Garland Thomson (New York: New York University Press, 1996), 208.

18   *Life of William Allen, with Selections from His Correspondence,* 3 vols. (London: Charles Gilpin, 1847), 46–47; cited in Hamblyn, 76.

19   Hamblyn, 76.

20   *Life of William Allen,* 1:57–61; cited in Hamblyn, 171.

21   John Stuart Mill, *Autobiography,* in *Prose of the Victorian Period,* ed. William E. Buckler (Boston: Houghton Mifflin, 1958), 291.

22   Mill, 292.

23   J. J. Moreau (de Tours), *La psychologie morbide* (Paris: Victor Masson, 1859), 53; cited in Drinka, 54.

24   Moreau, 109; cited in Drinka, 57.

25   Arthur Schopenhauer, *The World as Will and Representation,* trans. E. F. J. Payne (New York: Dover, 1966), 2:137–38.

26   Théodule Ribot, *The Psychology of Attention* (Chicago: Open Court, 1896), 3; cited in Jonathan Crary, *Suspensions of Perception: Attention, Spectacle, and Modern Culture* (Cambridge, MA: MIT Press, 2001), 47n99.

27   Wilkie Collins, *Heart and Science* (London: Chatto and Windus, 1883; reprinted, Ontario: Broadview Press, 1996), 45.

28   Collins to Mrs. Augustus Frederick Lehman (February 25, 1883), Harry Ransom Research Center; Austin, Texas; in Collins, 372.

29   Robert Louis Stevenson, *The Strange Case of Dr. Jekyll and Mr. Hyde and Other Tales of Terror* (London: Penguin, 2002), 55.

30   Gauchet and Swain, 35.

31   Andrew Scull, "The Fiction of Foucault's Scholarship," *TLS,* March 21, 2007; at http://tls.timesonline.co.uk/article/0,25347-2626687,00.html (accessed March 21, 2007).

32   Jennifer L. Fleissner, *Women, Compulsion, Modernity: The Moment of American Naturalism* (Chicago: University of Chicago Press, 2004), 9.

33   Fleissner, 61.

34   Charles Turner Thackrah, *The Effects of Arts, Trades, and Professions, and of Civic States and Habits of Living, on Health and Longevity* (London: Longmore, 1831); in Hunter and Macalpine, 826.

35 S. Weir Mitchell, *Lectures on Diseases of the Nervous System, Especially in Women* (Philadelphia: Lea Brothers, 1885), 57.

36 Mitchell, 266.

37 See Maria Frawley, *Invalidism and Identity in Nineteenth-Century Britain* (Chicago: University of Chicago Press, 2004); Janet Oppenheim's *"Shattered Nerves": Doctors, Patients, and Depression in Victorian England* (New York: Oxford University Press, 1991); and Vrettos.

38 Edward Shorter, *From Paralysis to Fatigue: A History of Psychosomatic Illness in the Modern Era* (New York: Free Press, 1992).

39 Edwin Ash, *Nerves and the Nervous* (London: Mills and Boone, 1911), 1–2.

CHAPTER FOUR

1 Frederick Brown, *Zola: A Life* (Baltimore: Johns Hopkins, 1995; reprinted 1996), 411.

2 Brown, 411.

3 Anthony Trollope, *An Autobiography* (London: Oxford University Press, 1923; reprinted 1936), 30.

4 Werner Muensterberger, *Collecting: An Unruly Passion* (Princeton, NJ: Princeton University Press, 1994), 119, 121.

5 Edward Bulwer-Lytton, *Confessions of a Water Patient* (London: H. Bailliere, 1848), 15.

6 Zola wrote nearly 1,700 articles for the journal *Le Semaphore de Marseille* before he published the first book of the Rougon-Macquart series (Brown, 397).

7 Of the studies undertaken of criminals, he cites his own work and that of Cesare Lombroso.

8 Émile Zola, *Thérèse Raquin,* trans. Leonard Tancock (New York: Penguin, 1962; reprinted 1978), 22.

9 Brown, 188.

10 Cited in Brown, 189.

11 Émile Zola, *The Experimental Novel and Other Essays,* trans. Belle M. Sherman (New York: Haskell House, 1964), 18.

12 Arthur MacDonald, *Émile Zola: A Study of His Personality* (Washington, DC, 1898), 468.

13 MacDonald, 468.

14 Émile Zola, *The Dreyfus Affair: "J'accuse" and Other Writings,* ed. Alain Pagès, trans. Eleanor Levieux (New Haven, Yale University Press, 1996), xiv.

15 See Steven Marcus, *Representations: Essays on Literature and Society* (New York: Columbia University Press, 1990), 56–91, for a discussion of Dora in relation to the novel.

16 MacDonald, 469.

17   Max Nordau, *Degeneration,* trans. Anonymous (New York: Appleton, 1895; reprinted Lincoln: University of Nebraska Press, 1993), 17.

18   Nordau, 18. As a sign of this obsession with books and writing, Flaubert wrote a short story called "Bibliomania" about a compulsive collector of books.

19   MacDonald, 478.

20   Nordau, 502.

21   MacDonald, 484.

22   Valentin Magnan, a psychiatrist who studied criminality and degeneracy, had written, "A hereditary degenerate could be a savant, a distinguished magistrate, a politician, an able administrator, and present from the moral point of view 'profound defects'" (translation mine). "Remarks at Meeting of Medico-Psychological Society, 27 July 1885," *Annales médico-psychologiques* 3 (1886), 99; cited in Daniel Pick, *Faces of Degeneration: A European Disorder, 1848–1918* (Cambridge: Cambridge University Press, 1989; reprinted 1996), 42n.

23   This also apparently accounts for Zola's preference to never reread his own books.

24   Steven Levenkron, *Obsessive-Compulsive Disorders: Treating and Understanding Crippling Habits* (New York: Time Warner, 1991); Judith L. Rappoport, *The Boy Who Couldn't Stop Washing* (New York: Signet, 1989); Marc Summers (with Eric Hollander), *Everything in Its Place: My Trials and Triumphs with Obsessive Compulsive Disorder* (London: Penguin, 1999; reprinted 2000).

25   See my "Dr. Johnson, Amelia, and the Discourse of Disability," in my *Bending Over Backwards,* 47–66.

26   MacDonald, 484.

27   MacDonald, 484.

28   Zola, Rougon-Macquart series, 4:1626; cited in Brown, 614.

29   Cited in Brown, 614.

30   Zola, *Masterpiece,* 41.

31   Brain or nerve lesions could be physical, visible lesions in the brain or on the nerves, or more abstractly a disorganization of nervous energy in general. See Arnold Davidson, *The Emergence of Sexuality: Historical Epistemology and the Formations of Concepts* (Cambridge: Harvard University Press, 2001), 2–29.

32   Zola, *Masterpiece,* 285.

33   Zola, *Thérèse Raquin,* 22–23.

34   Gustave Flaubert, *Bouvard and Pécuchet,* trans. A. J. Krailsheimer (London: Penguin, 1976), 24.

35   Gustave Flaubert, *Bibliomania* (London: Rodale Press, 1954), 14.

36   Flaubert, *Bouvard and Pécuchet,* 131.

37 Cited in Nicholas A. Basbanes, *A Gentle Madness: Bibliophiles, Bibliomanes, and the Eternal Passion for Books* (New York: Henry Holt, 1995), 27.

38 Thomas Frognall Dibdin, *Bibliomania; or, Book Madness: A Bibliographical Romance in Six Parts* (London: J. M. McCreery, 1811), 85.

39 Isaac D'Israeli, *Curiosities of Literature* (London: John Murray, 1807); cited in Dibdin, viii.

40 Dibdin, 13, 51.

41 Dibdin, 14.

42 Muensterberger, 74.

43 Muensterberger, 74.

44 A. N. L. Munby, "Only Collect: Portrait of an Obsession" (London: Maggs Bros., 2007), at http://www.maggs.com/collections/onlycollect.asp?book=17&page=3 (accessed February 2, 2007).

45 Muensterberger, 75.

46 Muensterberger, 97.

47 John Hill Burton, *The Book Hunter* (Philadelphia: Robert A. Tripple, 1881), 17.

CHAPTER FIVE

1 Helen Lefkowitz Horowitz, *Rereading Sex: Battles over Sexual Knowledge and Suppression in Nineteenth-Century America* (New York: Alfred A. Knopf, 2002), 5.

2 Horowitz's book amply illustrates this point. For further reading also see Lucy Bland and Laura Doan, eds., *Sexology Uncensored: The Documents of Sexual Science* (Chicago: University of Chicago Press, 1998); and Lucy Bland and Lara Doan, *Sexology in Culture: Labelling Bodies and Desires* (Cambridge: Polity Press, 1998; reprinted Chicago: University of Chicago Press, 1998).

3 Shorter, 56–58.

4 Cited in Shorter, 57.

5 "Advice to Doctors on Psychoanalytic Treatment" (1915), in *Wild Analysis*, ed. Adam Phillips, trans. Abel Bance (London: Penguin, 2002), 34.

6 Actually, Freud says specifically that "the *Ucs.* of one human being can react upon that of another, without passing through the *Cs.*" *SE* 14:194.

7 "Advice," 36.

8 Letter, May 16, 1900, in Sigmund Freud and Wilhelm Fliess, *The Complete Letters of Sigmund Freud to Wilhelm Fliess, 1887–1904*, ed. and trans. Jeffrey Masson (Cambridge, MA: Harvard University Press, 1985), 129.

9 Letter, May 16, 1900.

10 Cited in Peter Kramer, "Adirondack Couch," *New York Times Book Review*, December 24, 2006, 17.

11 Dan J. Stein, preface to Dan J. Stein and Michael H. Stone, *Essential Papers*

on Obsessive-Compulsive Disorder (New York: New York University Press, 1997), 1.

12   An interesting paradox arises. If neurasthenia was monotonous, then it was in a sense obsessional, since the repetition of the same thing might be defined as obsessional thinking. So we can speculate that rather than simply being monotonous, neurasthenia was more like the previous obsession, displaced by the newer one of the sexual etiology of anxiety neuroses.

13   Adam Phillips, *On Kissing, Tickling, and Being Bored* (London: Faber and Faber, 1993), 51.

14   Carl E. Schorske, "Artist of Angst," *New York Review of Books* 33 (January 15, 1987), 21–22.

15   And later, of course, Freud would combine anxiety and warfare in his essay on the death instinct in his *Beyond the Pleasure Principle* (*SE* 18:1–143).

16   It is worth noting that heredity requires that one be able to trace one's forebears—that one possess a traceable history. (Sir Francis Galton, for example, had one drawn up going back to the tenth century.) Such genealogies were not widely available to the poor, Jews, immigrants, and the like. Freud, rather than pin fate on lineage, favored an immediate, individual, and personal explanation of the problem. Obsession provided that immediate explanation.

17   Lydia Flem, *Freud the Man,* trans. Susan Fairfield (New York: Other Press, 2003), 104.

18   Flem, 104.

19   Sigmund Freud and Oskar Pfister, *Psycho-Analysis and Faith: The Letters of Sigmund Freud and Oskar Pfister,* ed. E. L. Freud and H. Meng, trans. E. Mosbacher (New York: Basic Books, 1963), 32–33; cited in Flem, 126.

20   Sigmund Freud and Lou Andréas-Salomé, *Sigmund Freud and Lou Andréas-Salomé.* Letters, ed. E Pfieffer, trans. W. Robson-Scott and E. Robson-Scott (New York: Norton, 1985) 51 cited in Flem, 126.

21   Louis Breger, *Freud: Darkness in the Midst of Vision* (New York: John Wiley, 2000), 67.

22   Wilhelm Stekel, *The Autobiography of Wilhelm Stekel,* ed. E. Guthel (New York: Liveright, 1950), 66; cited in Flem, 116.

23   A more recent translation uses the word "wretched" to describe his sex life. See Sigmund Freud, *The "Wolfman" and Other Cases,* trans. Louise Adey Huish (London: Penguin, 2002), 128.

24   Ernest Jones, *The Life and Work of Sigmund Freud,* vol. 2, *Years of Maturity, 1901–1939* (New York: Basic Books, 1955), 344; cited in Flem, 97.

25   Esquirol, 342ff.

26   David J. Lynn, "Sigmund Freud's Psychoanalysis of Albert Hirst," *Bulletin of the History of Medicine* 71:1 (1997), 69.

27 All of this confusion is further confused by the editors' note in the Standard Edition that "unfortunately the original map, printed in the German edition of 1924 and later, as well as in the English translation in Volume 3 of Freud's *Collected Papers* (p. 349), was itself totally inconsistent with some of the peculiar data presented in the case history. An entirely new one has been constructed for the present edition" (*SE* 10:212n1).

28 As a later psychoanalyst cautions, "It is inevitable that the therapist will occasionally get caught in the flypaper of the obsessional's way of life, and he must recognize it as quickly as possible so as to avoid as much of it as he can." Leonard Salzman, *Therapy of the Obsessive Personality* (New York: Jason Aronson, 1980); in Stein and Stone, 124.

29 See Patrick J. Mahoney, *Freud and the Rat Man* (New Haven: Yale University Press, 1986).

30 Interestingly, Anna Freud, in summarizing the special subject of the Twenty-Fourth International Psycho-Analytic Congress devoted to obsessional neurosis, said in 1966 of the focal point of obsession, "To say the least, it has presented us with a vivid picture of analytic problem-solving, with its painstaking back and forth between observation of clinical data, abstraction and generalization, and reapplication of theoretical thinking to the further elucidation of our patients' material." One can see in her language, perhaps, an echo of her father's continuing obsessional operations of psychoanalytic practice. Anna Freud, "Obsessional Neurosis: A Summary of Psycho-Analytic Views as Presented at the Conference," *International Journal of Psychoanalysis* 47 (1966), 122; in Stein and Stone, 112.

31 Gerald Graff, *Professing Literature: An Institutional History* (Chicago: University of Chicago Press, 1987), 56ff.

32 George Santayana, *Character and Opinion in the United States* (New York: Norton, 1967), 142; cited in Graff, 62.

CHAPTER SIX

1 Sullivan, 2.

2 Sullivan 4.

3 Theodoor H. Van de Velde, *Ideal Marriage: Its Physiology and Technique,* trans. Stella Browne (New York: Random House, 1936), 311.

4 For a detailed, although somewhat superficial account of the history of erotomania see G. E. Berrios and N. Kennedy, "Erotomania: A Conceptual History," *History of Psychiatry* 13 (2002), 381–400.

5 Carol Nealy, *Distracted Subjects: Madness and Gender in Shakespeare and Early Modern Culture* (Ithaca, NY: Cornell University Press, 2004), 99.

6   André Du Laurens, *A Discourse on the Preservation of the Sight: Of Melancholike Diseases,* trans. R. Surphlet (London: F. Kingston for R. Jacson, 1599); Shakespeare Association Facsimile 15, ed. S. V. Larkey and Humphrey Milford (Oxford: Oxford University Press, 1938); cited in Nealy, 102.

7   M.-D.-T. de Bienville, *La Nymphomanie ou traité de la fureur utérine* (Amsterdam: M. M. Rey) cited in Berrios and Kennedy, 386.

8   On this subject, in 1918 Maude Allen, a dancer of some note, was accused by member of Parliament Noel Pemberton-Billing of being part of a "cult of the clitoris," the implication being that she was a lesbian. See Lucy Bland, "Trial by Sexology? Maud Allan, *Salome,* and the 'Cult of the Clitoris' Case," in Bland and Doan, *Sexology and Culture,* 183–98.

9   For more than you ever wanted to know about masturbation, see Thomas Lacquer, *Solitary Sex: A Cultural History of Masturbation* (New York: Zone Books, 2003).

10   See Canguilhem.

11   The term "sexology" was coined, in German [as *Sexualwissenschaft*], by Iwan Bloch in 1907 in his book *The Sexual Life of Our Time.*

12   Davidson, 32.

13   Alice B. Stockham, *Karezza: Ethics of Marriage* (Chicago: Progress Company, 1903), 21.

14   See Patricia J. Campbell, *Sex Education Books for Young Adults, 1892–1979* (New York: Bowker, 1979).

15   B. G. Jefferis and J. L. Nichols, *Safe Counsel or Practical Eugenics* (Philadelphia: Domino Publishing, 1926), 74.

16   Steven Marcus's pioneering work *The Other Victorians* (New York: Basic Books, 1966) allows us to understand that the cliché of Victorian prudery was not necessarily the rule.

17   Jefferis, 203–4.

18   Van de Velde, 2.

19   One advertisement in the back of a marriage manual published in 1938 touts a book called *Love: A Treatise on the Science of Sex Attraction* in this way: "Because of the thoroughness and completeness of its contents and the minute details discussed in each chapter, the sale of this volume was formerly restricted to physicians. Now, however, this unusually valuable book has been made available to the general public." The crossover between physician reader and lay public is both descriptive and of course a selling point for the publishers.

20   Van de Velde, 24. Van de Velde tends to use italics in his writing, which I have preserved in the following quotations.

21   Interestingly, this same formulation can be made in the late twentieth century by sociologist Anthony Giddens: "The impulse to subordinate

and humiliate women . . . is probably a generic aspect of male psychology."
Giddens, *The Transformation of Intimacy: Sexuality, Love and Eroticism in Modern Societies* (Stanford: Stanford University Press, 1992), 121.

22 An interesting sea change from pre-nineteenth-century views in which the male represented rationality and the female irrationality in areas of sexuality.

23 Berrios and Kennedy, 397.

24 Cited in Bland and Doan, *Sexology Uncensored,* 130–31.

25 Marie Carmichael Stopes, *Married Love: A New Contribution to the Solution of Sex Difficulties* (New York: Eugenics Publishing Company, 1918; reprinted 1931), 5.

26 Again, compared to pre-nineteenth-century notions of female sexuality as rapacious, this new notion has to be seen in its historical context. Compare this to a line given to a female character in Catherine Breillat's 1999 film *Romance* who says matter-of-factly, "Everyone knows that women need more orgasms than men."

27 Stopes, 65, 76.

28 M. J. Exner, *The Sexual Side of Marriage* (New York: Eugenics Publishing Company, 1938), 72.

29 Stopes, 54.

30 Exner, 72.

31 Exner, 72; citing Knight Dunlap, *Social Psychology* (Baltimore: Williams and Wilkins, 1925), 41.

32 Exner, 90.

33 Janice M. Irvine, *Disorders of Desire: Sex and Gender in Modern American Sexology* (Philadelphia: Temple University Press, 1990), 46.

34 William H. Masters and Virginia E. Johnson, *Human Sexual Response* (New York: Little Brown, 1966), v.

35 Evelyn Millis Duvall, *Facts of Life and Love for Teenagers* (New York: Associated Press, 1950), 89.

36 Lois Pemberton, *The Stork Didn't Bring You!* (New York: Thomas Nelson and Sons, 1948). 18.

37 Pemberton, 20.

38 Eustace Chesser, *Love without Fear: How to Achieve Sex Happiness in Marriage* (New York: Signet, 1947), 90.

39 Chesser, 90.

40 Irvine, 98.

41 *SAR Guide for a Better Sex Life* (San Francisco: National Sex Forum, 1975), 15; cited in Irvine, 106.

42 And as long as local penal codes do not prohibit certain behaviors. For example, the well-publicized agreement between two men to have sex, then

have one man murder the other and eat him, clearly would violate even the most generous notion of consenting adults.

43 See Al Cooper, ed., *Sex and the Internet: A Guidebook for Clinicians* (New York: Brunner-Routledge, 2002).

44 Giddens, 74–75.

45 For a detailed history of this subject, see Richard Davenport-Hines, *The Pursuit of Oblivion: A Global History of Narcotics* (New York: Norton, 2002).

46 Interestingly, there has been a countermovement that wishes to correct the medicalization of a good deal of life. This movement includes people with disabilities, consumers of mental health services, homosexuals, people of color, and women—all of whom have been heavily medicalized and overstudied. But some of these groups are caught on the horns of a dilemma—would it be better for homosexuality to be a genetically de-termined set of behaviors? Will people of color wish to see themselves as genetically the same or different from the dominant white group because of health-care issues, traits and diseases relatively unique to them?

47 Peter Trachtenberg, *The Casanova Complex: Compulsive Lovers and Their Women* (London: Eden Books, 1988), 28.

48 Stanton Peele and Archie Brodsky, *Love and Addiction* (New York: Taplinger, 1975; reprinted London: Sphere Books, 1977), 27.

49 http://www.slaafws.org/FAQ.pdf (visited 6/17/06).

50 Peele and Brodsky, 13.

51 Giddens, 75.

52 John Money, *Love and Love Sickness: The Science of Sex, Gender Difference, and Pair-Bonding* (Baltimore: Johns Hopkins Press, 1980), 94.

53 There is some disagreement on whether you get to choose your sexual-ity or not. The ramifications of the freedom to choose are considerable. If you are homosexual, you might want to make sexual orientation not a matter of choice but of biology—that is, you might want to do this if you wish to show that homosexuality is "natural." On the other hand, if you are queer, you might want to emphasize that you actively chose a lifestyle and a way of life based on a political and cultural awareness. You don't want your choice relegated to biology. If you want to argue that sexual identity is shaped by sexist or paternalistic forces in society, you will want to indicate that one's sexuality is determined by the ideology of society. If you are transsexual, you may believe that your biological body is wrong and that you need to correct this by surgery and hormones. And if you are a brain scientist, you'll want to say that one's sexual proclivities are in the genes and the brain.

54 Trachtenberg, 18.

55 La Comtesse d'Albany, *Le Portfeuille . . .* (Paris: Pelissier, 1902); cited in

J. Rives Childs, *Casanoviana: An Annotated World Bibliography of Jacques Casanova de Seingalt and of Works Concerning Him* (Vienna: Nebehay, 1956), 218.

56 Heinrich Heine, "Briefe von Berlin," in *Werke,* ed. Elster, 7:593–94; cited in Childs, 285.

57 Theodor Mundt, *Madonna: Unterhaltungen mit einer Heiligen* (Leipzig, 1835); cited in Childs, 322.

58 [Anon.], *Allgemeine deutsche Real Encyclopädie* (Leipzig: Brockhaus, 1851), 373; cited in Childs, 219.

59 Masturbation was perhaps a different case in point. It was first critiqued in the eighteenth century, but it wasn't until Tissot's book in the nineteenth century that it came to be seen as a disease entity. However, its existence as a disease was predicated on the fact that it wasn't sexual intercourse. Intercourse was seen as healthful, while chastity was seen as a problem. See Laqueur's *Solitary Sex* for a much more detailed account.
Interestingly, Casanova was perhaps the model for Mozart's Don Juan. Don Juan and Casanova have been used interchangeably as templates for men who seduce women. But there is a dichotomy between the crassness of repeated seduction and the finesse and care that Casanova and Don Juan gave to the art of love, care that made them so irresistible to women and to the public eye. Havelock Ellis said of Casanova, he "loved many women but broke few hearts" (Havelock Ellis, *Psychology of Sex* [London: Heinemann, 1946], 189; cited in Giddens, 82). Van de Velde, the author of *Ideal Marriage,* recommends Don Juan as a model to his male readers: "The soul of this arch lover was not seeking the base triumph of snatching and throwing away, but ever and only the ecstasy of giving the joy of love. And in this sense the husband should act the part of Don Juan to his wife over again. Then, in giving delight, he will himself experience it anew and permanently, and his marriage will become *ideal*" (Van de Velde, 126).

60 Peele and Brodsky, 14.

61 Pia Mellody, *Facing Love Addiction: Giving Yourself the Power to Change the Way You Love* (New York: HarperCollins, 1992), viii.

62 Peele and Brodsky, 16.

63 Mellody, 225.

64 *Sex and Love Addicts Anonymous* (Boston: Augustine Fellowship, 1986), vii.

65 *Sex and Love Addicts Anonymous,* vi.

66 Peele and Brodsky, 18.

67 Trachtenberg, 201.

68 S. C. Kalichman, J. R. Johnson, V. Adair, D. Rompa, K. Multhauf, and J. A. Kelly, "Sexual Sensation Seeking: Scale Development and Predicting AIDS-risk Behavior among Homosexually Active Men," *Journal of Personality Assessment* 62 (1994), 385–97. It is worth noting that this com-

monly used scale to measure sexual compulsivity was developed in order to predict homosexual activity in the context of AIDS.

69 J. P. Schneider, "Sex addiction: Controversy within Mainstream Addiction Medicine, Diagnosis Based on the DSV-III-R and Physician Case Histories," *Sexual Addiction and Compulsivity* 1 (1994), 19–44.

70 Holly Fahner, "Is There a Casanova Gene?" *Glamour,* June 2006, 138.

71 S. Gold and C. Hefner, "Many Conceptions, Minimal Data," *Clinical Psychology Review* 18:3 (1998), 367–81.

72 Giddens, 49–64.

73 Exner, 71.

74 Erich Fromm, *The Art of Loving* (New York: Harper and Row, 1956; reprinted New York: Bantam, 1963).

75 Fromm, 73.

76 Christopher Lasch, *Haven in a Heartless World: The Family Besieged* (New York: Norton, 1995).

77 Fromm, 81–83.

78 Fromm, 92.

79 *Sex and Love Addicts Anonymous,* viii.

80 Mellody, 7.

81 Nicholas Bakalar, "Review Sees No Advantage in 12-Step Programs," *New York Times,* July 25, 2006, F6.

82 Craig Nakken, *The Addictive Personality: Understanding Compulsion in Our Lives* (New York: Harper and Row, 1988), 26.

83 J. Reid Meloy, *The Psychology of Stalking* (San Diego: Academic Press, 1998), xix.

84 J. R. Meloy and H. Fisher, "Some Thoughts on the Neurobiology of Stalking," *Forensic Science* 50:6 (November 2005): 1472–80.

85 Richard Gallagher, *I'll Be Watching You: True Stories of Stalkers and Their Victims* (London: Virgin, 2001), 15.

86 Meloy, 2.

87 Meloy, 13–14.

88 Esquirol, 347; cited in Berrios and Kennedy, 389.

89 Berrios and Kennedy, 390.

90 Bénédict Morel, *Études cliniques: Traité théorique et pratique des maladies mentales* (Paris: Masson, 1853), 2:256; cited in Berrios and Kennedy, 390.

91 Vladimir Nabokov, *Lolita* (New York: Vintage, 1991), 9.

92 Nabokov, 88.

93 Cited in A. M. Homes, *The End of Alice* (New York: Scribner's, 1996), i.

94 Jeffrey Rosen, "The Brain on the Stand: How Neuroscience Is Transforming the Legal System," *New York Times Magazine,* March 11, 2007, 52.

95 Rosen, 53.

CHAPTER SEVEN

1   http://art-bin.com/art/klingertexts/klinger.html.

2   J. Kirk T. Varnedoe, *Graphic Works of Max Klinger* (New York: Dover, 1977), xiii–xiv.

3   Peter Schjeldahl, "The Far Side: An Outsider Artist's Scary Grandeur," *New Yorker,* May 5, 2003; http://www.newyorker.com/critics/art/?030505craw_artworld.

4   Schjeldahl.

5   Adams, 220.

6   Schjeldahl.

7   Jane Green and Leah Levy, eds., *Jay DeFeo and "The Rose."* (Berkeley: University of California Press, 2003), ix.

8   While the museum usually becomes the space in which work on a canvas comes to an end—the equivalent in a sense of publication—DeFeo could not allow that limit to apply. In this sense, she parallels the other early obsessive painter, J. M. W. Turner, who was said to have painted his works while they were on salon walls so that his colors might outshine those of the adjacent paintings.

9   *A Thousand Plateaus: Capitalism and Schizophrenia* (Minneapolis: University of Minnesota Press, 1987), 9.

10 Robert Hobbs, ed., *Mark Lombardi: Global Networks* (New York: Independent Curators International, 2003), 33.

11 http://www.pierogi2000.com/memorial/lombardm.html.

12 Ken Johnson, "Mark Lombardi: Vicious Circles," *New York Times,* November 5, 1999, E 41.

13 Hobbs, 51.

14 http://www.steamshovelpress.com/altmedia18.html.

15 http://www.almartinraw.com.

16 http://www.almartinraw.com.

17 http://www.pierogi2000.com/memorial/lombardm.html.

18 http://www.prisonplanet.com/articles/december2004/131204commitssuicide.htm.

19 Elisa Longhauser and Elka Spoerri, *The Other Side of the Moon: The World of Adolf Wölfli* (Philadelphia: Goldie Paley Gallery; Moore College of Art, 1988), 35.

CHAPTER EIGHT

1   Michael A. Jenike, Lee Baer, and William E. Minichiello, *Obsessive-Compulsive Disorders: Practical Management* (New York: Mosby, 1998), 4. Adams, 17.

2   Adams, 17.

3   Eric Hollander, "Obsessive-Compulsive Disorder: The Hidden Epidemic," *Journal of Clinical Psychiatry* 58, suppl. 12 (1997), 4.

4   *Mental Health: A Call for Action by World Health Ministers* (Geneva: World Health Organization, 2001), 16.

5   Jenike et al., xvi.

6   See for example Barbara Herrnstein Smith, *Scandalous Knowledge: Science, Truth, and the Human* (Durham, NC: Duke University Press, 2005); or Donna Haraway, *Modest_Witness@Second Millennium* (New York: Routledge, 1997).

7   Michael Stone, introduction to Stein and Stone, 23–24.

8   Rasmussen and Eisen, in Jenike et al., 31.

9   Adams, 9–10.

10 Myrna M. Weissman, Roger C. Bland, et al., "The Cross National Epidemiology of Obsessive Compulsive Disorder," *Journal of Clinical Psychiatry* 55:3 (supplement) (March 1994), 5–10.

11 Rasmussen and Eisen, in Jenike et al., 25.

12 Rasmussen and Eisen, in Jenike et al., 16.

13 S. Rachman and P. DeSilva, "Abnormal and Normal Obsessions," *Behavior Research Therapy* 16:4 (1978), 233–48.

14 J. H. Greist, J. W. Jefferson, K. A. Kobak, et al., "Efficacy and Tolerability of Serotonin Transport Inhibitors in Obsessive Compulsive Disorder," *Archives of General Psychiatry* 52:1 (1995), 53–60

15 M. M. Weissman, R. C. Bland, G. J. Canino et al., "The Cross-National Epidemiology of Obsessive-Compulsive Disorder," *Journal of Clinical Psychology* 55, suppl. 3 (1994), 10.

16 Not that this hasn't been tried. Most recently in Brian Knutson, Scott Rick, G. Elliott Wimmer, Drazen Prelec, and George Loewenstein, "Neural Predictors of Purchases," *Neuron* 53:1 (January 4, 2007), 147–56; or Dharol Tankersley, C. Jill Stowe, and Scott A. Huettel, "Altruism Is Associated with an Increased Neural Response to Agency," *Nature Neuroscience;* published online, January 21, 2007, at http://www.nature.com/neuro/journal/vaop/ncurrent/abs/nn1833.html.

17 While there is much enthusiasm in trying to establish a genetic basis for OCD and other mental disorders, that process needs greater scrutiny. The general method of doing this is enhanced by computer technologies that allow a great computing power to scan massive numbers of SNPs. However, the ease with which this can be done permits a kind of sloppy science that coordinates any set of SNPs with any set of disorders.

18 Freud himself wrote that "sufferers from this illness are consequently able to treat their affliction as a private matter and keep it concealed for many years. And, indeed, many more people suffer from these forms of obses-

sional neurosis that doctors hear of. For many sufferers, too concealment is made easier from the fact that they are quite well able to fulfil their social duties during a part of the day, once they have devoted a number of hours to their secret doings." *SE* 9:119. Of course, there is a major problem with what Freud says, since how would it be possible for him to know what it is that doctors do not hear of? In addition, the supposition is that the neurosis is minor enough to conceal it from friends and family, and that a person of ordinary means would have a large amount of time for rituals apart from the fulfilling of their social obligations.

19 For example, Rachman et al. note that "obsessive-compulsive disorders are so distressing to patients and their families." Stanley Rachman, Ray Hodgson, and Isaac M. Marks, "The Treatment of Obsessive-Compulsive Neurosis," *Behavior Research and Therapy* 9 (1971); cited in Stein and Stone, 203.

20 H. Gilbert Welch, Lisa Schwartz, and Steven Woloshin, "What's Making Us Sick Is an Epidemic of Diagnoses," *New York Times,* January 2, 2007, F5.

21 Among others see David Healy, *Let Them Eat Prozac: The Unhealthy Relationship between the Pharmaceutical Industry and Depression* (New York: NYU Press, 2004); his *The Creation of Psychopharmacology* (Cambridge, MA: Harvard University Press, 2004); and Meika Loe, *The Rise of Viagra: How the Little Blue Pill Changed Sex in America* (New York: NYU Press, 2004). Christopher Lane, *Shyness: How Normal Behavior Became a Sickness* (New Haven: Yale University Press, 2007).

22 Adams, 209.

23 Carl Elliott and Peter D. Kramer *Better Than Well: American Medicine Meets the American Dream* (New York: Norton, 2003). In a recent lecture, Carl Elliott pointed out that these ghostwritten articles are placed in better and more prestigious journals than those written by ordinary researchers. Further, such articles are cited at least 50 percent more often than other articles (lecture at "Against Health" conference, University of Michigan School of Medicine, November 2007). See also David Healy and Dinah Cattell, "Interface between Authorship, Industry, and Science in the Domain of Therapeutics," *British Journal of Psychiatry* 8:3 (2003), 1, 22–27.

24 Eric Hollander, foreword to Summers, xv.

25 http://www.medscape.com/viewarticle/507104 (accessed January 5, 2007).

26 Gardiner Harris and Janet Roberts, "A State's Files Put Doctors' Ties to Drug Makers on Close View," *New York Times,* March 21, 2007, A1, A19.

27 Jenike, in Stein and Stone, 304.

28 http://www.mclean.harvard.edu/pdf/about/bios/cv-mjenike.pdf (accessed March 30, 2007).

29 Gardiner Harris, "FDA Limits Role of Advisers Tied to Industry," *New*

York Times, March 22, 2007; http://www.nytimes.com/2007/03/22/ washington/22fda.html (accessed March 27, 2007).

30 Hollander, *Obsessive-Compulsive Disorder,* 4.

31 Rapoport, 13, 8.

32 Lee Baer, *Getting Control: Overcoming Your Obsessions and Compulsions* (Boston: Little, Brown, and Company, 1991), 5.

33 Gail Steketee and Teresa Pigott, *Obsessive Compulsive Disorder: The Latest Assessment and Treatment Strategies* (Kansas City, MO: Compact Clinicals, 1999), 1.

34 *New England Journal of Medicine* 321:8 (1989), 539–41.

35 Hollander, "Obsessive-Compulsive Disorder," 3–6.

36 See for example Allan V. Horwitz and Jerome C. Wakefield, *The Loss of Sadness: How Psychiatry Transformed Normal Sorrow into Depressive Disorder* (New York: Oxford University Press, 2007).

37 Paul Daniel Arnold, Tricia Sicard, Eliza Burroughs, Margaret A. Richter, and James L. Kennedy, "Glutamate Transporter Gene *SLC1A1* Associated with Obsessive-Compulsive Disorder," *Archives of General Psychiatry* 63 (2006), 776.

38 Diane E. Dickel, Jeremy Veenstra-VanderWeele, Nancy J. Cox, Xiaolin Wu, Daniel J. Fischer, Michelle Van Etten-Lee, Joseph A. Himle, Bennett L. Leventhal, Edwin H. Cook Jr., and Gregory L. Hanna, "Association Testing of the Positional and Functional Candidate Gene *SLC1A1/ EAAC1* in Early-Onset Obsessive-Compulsive Disorder," *Archives of General Psychiatry* 63 (2006), 785.

39 Summers, 55.

40 Erick H. Turner, Annette M. Matthews, Eftihia Linardatos, Robert A. Tell, and Robert Rosenthal, "Selective Publication of Antidepressant Trials and Its Influence on Apparent Efficacy," *New England Journal of Medicine* 358:3 (January 17, 2008), 252–60.

41 L. Kirsch, B. J. Deacon, T. B. Huedo-Medina, A. Scoboria, T. J. Moore et al., "Initial Severity and Antidepressant Benefits: A Meta-analysis of Data Submitted to the Food and Drug Administration," *PLoS Med* 5:2 (2008): e45; doi:10.1371/journal.pmed.0050045.

42 Rapoport, 12.

43 Joseph Zohar and Thomas R. Insel, "Obsessive-Compulsive Disorder: Psychobiological Approaches to Diagnosis, Treatment, and Pathophysiology," *Biological Psychiatry* 22 (1987), 687.

44 Knutson et al., 147–56.

45 L. R. Baxter, J. M. Schwartz, and K. S. Bergman, "Caudate Glucose Metabolic Rate Changes with Both Drug and Behavior Therapy for Obsessive-Compulsive Disorder," *Archives of General Psychiatry* 49 (1994), 681–89, as referenced by www.mental-health.com.

46 C. Benkelfat, T. E. Nordahl, W. E. Semple, A. C. King, D. L. Murphy, and R. M. Cohen, "Local Cerebral Glucose Metabolic Rates in Obsessive-Compulsive Disorder: Patients Treated with Clomipramine," *Archives of General Psychiatry* 47:9 (September 1990).

47 Stefan Ursu, V. Andere Stenger, M. Katherine Shear, Mark R. Jones, and Cameron S. Carter, "Overactive Action Monitoring in Obsessive-Compulsive Disorder: Evidence from Functional Magnetic Resonance Imaging," *Psychological Science* 14:4 (July 2003), 347.

48 Examples abound, but Barry R. Kamisaruck and Beverly Whipple, "Functional MRI of the Brain during Orgasm in Women," http://psychology .rutgers.edu/-brk/published051106.pdf (accessed January 22, 2007), might serve.

49 Mario Beauregard and Vincent Paquette, "Neural Correlates of a Mystical Experience in Carmelite Nuns," http://www.sciencedirect.com.proxy .cc.uic.edu/science?_ob=ArticleURL&_udi=B6T0G-4KGX8FB-1&_ user=186797&_coverDate=09%2F25%2F2006&_alid=529540678&_ rdoc=1&_fmt=full&_orig=search&_cdi=4862&_sort=d&_docanchor=& view=c&_ct=1&_acct=C000013678&_version *Neuroscience Letters* 405:3 (September 25, 2006), 186–90.

50 Y. Moriguchi et al., "Empathy and Judging Other's Pain: An fMRI Study of Alexithymia," *Cerebral Cortex* (advanced online publication December 5, 2006) http://cercor.oxfordjournals.org/cgi/content/abstract/bhl130v1 (accessed January 22, 2007).

51 Joshua D. Greene et al., "An fMRI Investigation of Emotional Engagement in Moral Judgment," *Science* 293:5537 (September 14, 2001), 2105–8.

52 Dennis Overbye, "Free Will: Now You Have It, Now You Don't," *New York Times,* January 2, 2007, F1.

53 John Schwartz, "Of Gay Sheep, Modern Science, and the Perils of Bad Publicity," *New York Times,* January 25, 2007, A20.

54 Alison McCook, "Is Peer Review Broken?" *Scientist* 20:2 (January 7, 2007), 26.

55 Gilbert Pinard, "The Pharmacologic and Psychological Treatment of Obsessive-Compulsive Disorder," *Canadian Journal of Psychiatry* 51:7 (June 2006), 405.

56 Pierre Blier, Kami Habib, and Martine F. Flament, "Pharmacotherapies in the Management of Obsessive-Compulsive Disorder," *Canadian Journal of Psychiatry* 51:7 (June 2006), 423.

57 Christo Todorov, Mark H. Freeston, and Francois Borgeat, "On the Pharmacotherapy of Obsessive-Compulsive Disorder: Is a Consensus Possible?" *Canadian Journal of Psychiatry* 45:3 (April 2000), 257–62.

58 Emily Colas, *Just Checking: Scenes from the Life of an Obsessive-Compulsive* (New York: Washington Square Press, 1998), 138.

59   Summers, 55.

60   Summers, 183, 188.

61   See G. Thomas Couser, *Recovering Bodies: Illness, Disability, and Life Writing* (Madison: University of Wisconsin Press, 1997).

62   Summers, 197.

63   Summers, 204.

64   Ian Osborn, *Tormenting Thoughts and Secret Rituals: The Hidden Epidemic of Obsessive-Compulsive Disorder* (New York: Pantheon, 1998), 71, 5.

65   Rapoport, 94.

66   http://www.ocfoundation.org/UserFiles/File/ITP_Interviews/Rosalind-Franklin-University.pdf (accessed January 29, 2007).

67   http://www.ocfoundation.org/dld/itp0002.pdf (accessed January 29, 2007).

68   http://www.ocfoundation.org/dld/itp0011.pdf (accessed January 29, 2007).

CHAPTER NINE

1   Lennard Davis and David Morris, "Biocultures Manifesto," *NLH* 38:3 (Summer 2007), 411–18.

2   Charles Anderson and Marian MacCurdy, *Writing and Healing: Toward an Informed Practice* (Urbana, IL: National Council of Teachers of English, 2001); Gillie Bolton, *Reflective Practice: Writing and Professional Development* (London: Paul Chapman Publishing, 2001); Cathy Caruth, *Unclaimed Experience: Trauma, Narrative, and History* (Baltimore: Johns Hopkins University Press, 1996); Rita Charon, "Narrative Medicine: A Model for Empathy, Reflection, Profession, and Trust," *Journal of the American Medical Association* 286 (2001): 1897–902. Shoshana Felman and Dori Laub, *Testimony: Crises of Witnessing in Literature, Psychoanalysis, and History* (New York: Routledge, 1992); Arthur Frank, *The Wounded Storyteller: Body, Illness, and Ethics* (Chicago: University of Chicago Press, 1995); Anne Hunsaker Hawkins, *Reconstructing Illness: Studies in Pathography,* 2nd ed. (West Lafayette, IN: Purdue University Press, 1999); Anne Hunsaker Hawkins and Marilyn Chandler McEntyre, *Teaching Literature and Medicine* (New York: Modern Language Association, 2000); Terrence Holt, "Narrative Medicine and Negative Capability," *Literature and Medicine* 23 (2004): 318–33. Kathryn Montgomery Hunter, *Doctors' Stories: The Narrative Structure of Medical Knowledge* (Princeton: Princeton University Press, 1991); Arthur Kleinman, *The Illness Narratives: Suffering, Healing, and the Human Condition* (New York: Basic Books, 1988); Shlomith Rimmon-Kenan, "The Story of 'I': Illness and Narrative Identity," *Narrative* 10 (2002): 9–27. Richard Zaner, *Conversations on the Edge: Narratives of Ethics and Illness* (Washington, DC: Georgetown University Press, 2004).

3   Rita Charon, "Narrative Medicine: Attention, Representation, Affilia-
      tion," *Narrative* 13.3 (2005), 261–70; at http://muse.jhu.edu/journals/
      narrative/v013/13.3charon.html (accessed February 23, 2007).
4   Bradley Lewis, "Reading Cultural Studies of Medicine," *Journal of Medical
      Humanities* 19.1 (Spring 1998), 9–24.
5   Felicia Aull, "Telling and Listening: Constraints and Opportunities," *Nar-
      rative* 13:3 (October 2005), 290.
6   Rachman, 15.

Index